Hearing Assistive and Access Technology

Hearing Assistive and Access Technology

Samuel R. Atcherson, PhD
Clifford A. Franklin, PhD
Laura Smith-Olinde, PhD

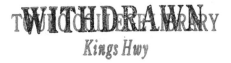
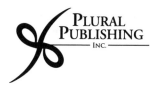
PLURAL
PUBLISHING
INC.

KH

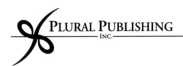

PLURAL PUBLISHING
INC.

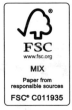

5521 Ruffin Road
San Diego, CA 92123

e-mail: info@pluralpublishing.com
Website: http://www.pluralpublishing.com

Typeset in 11/14 Minion Pro by Flanagan's Publishing Services, Inc.
Printed in the United States of America by McNaughton & Gunn, Inc.

Library of Congress Cataloging-in-Publication Data

Atcherson, Samuel R., author.
  Hearing assistive and access technology / Samuel R. Atcherson, Clifford A. Franklin, Laura
Smith-Olinde.
      p. ; cm.
  Includes bibliographical references and index.
  ISBN 978-1-59756-512-7 (alk. paper) — ISBN 1-59756-512-1 (alk. paper)
  I. Franklin, Clifford A., author. II. Smith-Olinde, Laura, author. III. Title.
  [DNLM: 1. Hearing Aids. 2. Hearing Loss—rehabilitation. 3. Communication Aids for
Disabled. 4. Correction of Hearing Impairment—methods. WV 274]
  RF300
  617.8'9—dc23
                    2014043383

2/3/16

Contents

Foreword

Drs. Atcherson, Franklin, and Smith-Olinde have written a *must-read* book about assistive and emerging technologies that can vastly increase the ability of consumers with hearing loss to hear more clearly, communicate more effectively, and enhance their quality of life. Although written primarily for hearing health care professionals, consumers, family members, and those who interact with people with hearing loss can greatly benefit from understanding how technology, beyond and in conjunction with hearing aids and implantable devices, can provide greater access to more opportunities.

Today there are 48 million Americans, nearly 20% of the population, who have a hearing loss. It is the third largest public health issue, after heart disease and arthritis, and the third most common chronic disability affecting older adults. With millions of baby boomers reaching their golden years and more young people, including one-in-four teens, with a hearing loss, these assistive technologies can provide immediate life-changing communication tools that benefit consumers of all ages and backgrounds.

At the Hearing Loss Association of America, the nation's largest organiza-tion for consumers with hearing loss, the overwhelming number of inquiries and issues surround the lack of knowledge and training about assistive and emerging technologies from hearing health care providers. We know from experience that consumers who use new and emerging technologies in conjunction with their hearing aids and implants can remove impediments to communication and hearing. To communicate, one must be able to understand and interpret sounds properly, to understand speech and be able to extract information, and to react appropriately to what is being said and what is happening—which is why assistive and emerging technologies are so important to consumers with hearing loss. These technologies do not work in isolation but work as part of an individual's communication system providing a more holistic approach to treatment.

The authors effectively highlight the power of harnessing new technology for better hearing, removing impediments, and training hearing health care professionals about the possibilities for consumers with hearing loss, not the limitations.

—Anna Gilmore Hall, RN, MS, CAE
Executive Director
Hearing Loss Association of
   America
Bethesda, Maryland

Preface

This book was conceived out of frustration for the lack of a current text of hearing assistive and access technologies. In our interaction with colleagues, students, and patients, we became increasingly aware of the lack of awareness, knowledge, and understanding of many powerful technologies available for individuals with hearing loss. It is quite unfortunate when the remediation of hearing loss stops with the fitting of hearing aids and implantable devices. These devices, while amazing, cannot solve every communication and access need. For individuals to be fully independent and have the opportunity for the highest quality of life possible, professionals and consumers alike need to begin thinking routinely and consistently beyond hearing aids and implantable devices. We need to better understand the rights of those with disabilities and be willing to examine a patient's life more holistically by understanding the patient's needs inside and outside the home. Technology is accelerating quickly and is evolving continually, that, admittedly, it is hard to keep up. But with basic foundational information and understanding, we can better imagine the possibilities and know where to look.

When we began the book, we realized very quickly what a daunting road we would have ahead of us. Hearing assistive and access technologies do not always fit neatly into discrete categories. Today, we see more cross-compatibility, interoperability, and merging of one or more technologies than ever before. The level of sophistication of those technologies is ever changing and becoming more advanced in speed and processing. Technologies designed for individuals with hearing loss may be beneficial for those without hearing loss, and vice versa. With technology, we appear to be approaching a form of technological universalism. We are excited about this possible future, but until we get there, we feel a significant responsibility to educate about existing technologies to create better opportunities for individuals with hearing loss.

It is our hope that those who choose (or are required) to read this book will have their eyes open to hearing assistive and access technologies, both old and new, and share in our passion for a better world for individuals with hearing loss. We simply need to stop living in the past with our preconceived limitations, and instead keep an open mind and an eye toward equal opportunity and equal access. Although no one can guarantee equal outcomes, failure to try could be the demise of the world as we know it. Thank you for your consideration in joining us on this journey.

—Samuel R. Atcherson,
Clifford A. Franklin, and
Laura Smith-Olinde

Acknowledgments

There are many heroes in the field of audiology and related fields who forged our interest and path for this book. A list of these heroes would be unnecessarily long and never ending, and we would likely inadvertently leave someone out in the process. Among these heroes are inventors, trailblazers, advocates, scientists, faculty, clinicians, rehabilitationists, educators, engineers, lobbyists, entrepreneurs, consumerists, and, of course, the individuals with hearing loss who are quite diverse. We thank each of you for your contribution in making this world a better place for individuals with hearing loss.

To complete this book, we knew we would not be able to do this alone. We have had our ups and downs and victories and shortcomings, all while managing, the best we could, our personal and professional lives with a variety of commitments, job changes, and family demands. For all these reasons, and many more, we thank the following individuals for their assistance in various phases of the project: Mary "Ish" Crigler, Julia Fitzer, Carrie Foley, Rachel Huber, Hillary Jones, Andrea Knapp, Meredith Levisee, Charlotte "Carly" Murry, Holly Myers, Taryn Pegram, Lindsey Sloan, Anna Westling, Rachel Weyrens, and McKenna Wright. Some of these individuals helped us in the earlier planning stages and resource gathering, while others helped us reach closure through editing, making helpful suggestions, helping with organization, and completing the glossary. We appreciate each of you very much, and we are pleased to have brought you into this project.

Finally, writing a book is a sacrificial effort. As authors, we sacrificed our personal and professional time, but those who were most affected were our family and friends who also made great sacrifices to allow us to continue to work on this book to fruition. We will never get that time back, but because of your sacrifice, we can try to make up for it in the coming months and years. We are truly grateful to our families who paid the price so that we might help individuals around the world with hearing loss. Thank you especially to Rebecca, Calleigh, and Bayleigh Atcherson (Sam's spouse and daughters); Ruth and Kenneth Zellmer (Sam's in-laws); Frank Olinde (Laura's spouse); and Jennifer and Meghan Franklin (Cliff's spouse and daughter). In addition, Cliff would like to acknowledge Jennifer, Clay, Alan, and Janelle Franklin, as audiologists and family. Thank you, and we love you.

*We dedicate this book to
our spouses, Rebecca, Jennifer, and Frank;
our children, Calleigh, Bayleigh, and Meghan;
and
our academic mentors, faculty colleagues,
and undergraduate and graduate students with whom we have worked
over the course of our careers.*

PART I

Fundamental Considerations

1

Introduction

Why Did We Write This Book?

As audiologists in the field of communication sciences and disorders, we believe in the inherent right of all individuals to be able to communicate with others, and we believe that all individuals have a right to equal access to information, education, enjoyment, and entertainment. We recognize, however, that there may never be equal outcomes. For individuals with disabilities, including communication disorders, we agree with the National Joint Committee for the Communication Needs of Persons with Severe Disabilities (NJC) who advocate the right to affect, through communication, the conditions of their existence. The NJC created and published a *Communication Bill of Rights* for all people with disabilities regardless of the extent or severity (NJC, 1992). The

Communication Bill of Rights states that each person has the right to:

- request desired objects, actions, events, and people;
- refuse undesired objects, actions, or events;
- express personal preferences and feelings;
- be offered choices and alternatives;
- reject offered choices;
- request and receive another person's attention and interaction;
- ask for and receive information about changes in routine and environment;
- receive intervention to improve communication skills;
- receive a response to any communication, whether or

3

not the responder can fulfill the request;

- have access to AAC (augmentative and alternative communication) and other AT (assistive technology) services and devices at all times;
- have AAC and other AT devices that function properly at all times;
- be in environments that promote one's communication as a full partner with other people, including peers;
- be spoken to with respect and courtesy;
- be spoken to directly and not be spoken for or talked about in the third person while present; and
- have clear, meaningful, and culturally and linguistically appropriate communications.

This book was conceived as part of our beliefs in these rights. For individuals with hearing loss, there continues to be injustice in terms of access to auditory information, and there continues to be a lack of awareness about various hearing assistive and access technologies. Because of hearing loss, some technologies have been developed to take advantage of other sensory functions, such as the eyes and tactile responses through our skin and body. In this book, we define hearing *assistive* technology as any device that helps to overcome hearing loss whether it is to provide or enhance sound, or to provide sound-based information in an alternative modality such as a visual or tactile cue. Hearing aids and implantable devices, however, are not considered directly under this definition but may well be used in conjunction with hearing assistive devices. We define hearing *access* technology as an approach to using devices to provide equal access and equal opportunity, but an approach that cannot guarantee equal outcomes. The term *access* is important here, since hearing aids, implantable devices, and various hearing assistive devices may help in some situations but not all.

One important consideration is that some of these technologies are used on a personal level, whereas others are used on a public level. A second important consideration is that the financial and maintenance responsibility for these technologies will vary considerably. A final important consideration is that not all assistive and access approaches are electronics based and may involve human and animal facilitators. We would hope that effective hearing assistive and access technologies together can enrich the lives of many individuals with hearing loss. By increasing awareness and promoting advocacy, this outcome is achievable.

Certainly, it does not help matters that there is a large inventory of hearing assistive and access technologies constantly evolving while new technologies continue to be developed. In spite of the large inventory, there remain some compatibility and interoperability concerns for some technologies, and these issues can lead to confusion that increases anxiety, frustration, incompetence, noncompliance, and wasted resources. Figure 1–1 offers a glimpse of how various wireless assistive technologies and their location on the electromagnetic spectrum (e.g., infrared [IR], near-field communication [NFC], frequency modulation [FM], digital enhanced cordless telecommunications [DECT], and Bluetooth) can feed into some of this confusion. We hope this book will reduce confusion and help educate and promote various hearing assistive and access technologies. However, we want to caution here that this book is not a user's guide for these technologies. Rather, we introduce or remind the reader about the existence of these technologies and offer examples and scenarios that help the reader understand situations in which that particular technology might be useful.

We believe this book will be helpful for a variety of individuals: audiologists,

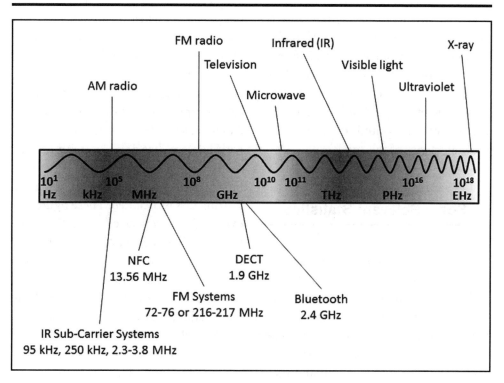

Figure 1–1. Various frequency bands on the electromagnetic spectrum. From left to right, the wavelengths progressively decrease, while frequencies increase. On the top of the figure are commonly recognized electromagnetic waves. On the bottom of the figure are transmission bands used by various communication devices and hearing assistive technologies. Abbreviations: *AM* = amplitude modulation; *FM* = frequency modulation; *IR* = infrared; *NFC* = near-field communication; *DECT* = digital enhanced cordless telecommunications; *Hz* = hertz (cycles/second); *k* = kilo; *M* = mega; *G* = giga; *T* = tera; *P* = peta; *E* = exa.

speech-language pathologists, special educators, school-based administrators, vocational rehabilitationists, consumerists, parents, and any individual experiencing hearing loss. This book was written in large part with first-year audiology graduate students in mind. In doing so, we aim to reach the most people possible to try to make a difference in the lives of individuals with hearing loss, their families, coworkers, and social spheres in a variety of settings. Although there is much information in this book, it is neither all-encompassing nor comprehensive. That was never the goal. Rather, it is intended as a starting place. Before we describe how to get the most out of this book, a review of some hearing loss statistics is helpful to get "the lay of the land," appreciate the magnitude of the issue, and the importance of this book.

Some Relevant Statistics

Hearing loss is a common disorder with a variety of congenital (present at birth) and acquired causes. In this brief section, we describe some relevant statistics pertaining to hearing loss. These statistics are helpful and necessary to understand the importance of early detection and intervention, accurate and timely diagnosis, personal and societal burden, treatment, and hearing loss prevention. Hearing loss that is not resolved, limits one or more daily activities, and/or restricts participation, is a serious issue, particularly when it negatively impacts communication and overall quality of life.

According to the World Health Organization (2012), an estimated 360 million individuals around the world (5.3% of the world population) have some form of debilitating hearing loss. Hearing loss is commonly cited as one of the top 10 disabilities in the United States (Kirshman & Grandgenett, 1997; U.S. Census Bureau, 2005), and the Better Hearing Institute (BHI) estimated that untreated hearing loss has economic impact in excess of $100 billion (Kochkin, 2005). This equates to a loss of up to $30,000 per person with hearing loss in lost salary and wages annually. With few exceptions, hearing loss can lead to lost productivity as well. For the U.S. population ages 12 years and up, Lin, Niparko, and Ferrucci (2011) reported an estimated 30 million Americans (12.7% of the U.S. population) with bilateral hearing loss, with an estimated increase to 48.1 million Americans (20.3% of the population) when unilateral hearing loss is included. These figures are expected to grow because of the aging population (Lin et al., 2011), the increase in childhood noise exposure (Niskar et al., 2001) and noise exposure, smoking, and various cardiovascular risks of young adults (Agrawal, Platz, & Niparko, 2008; Le Prell, Hensley, Campbell, Hall, & Guire, 2011). Approximately 15% of Americans (26 million) between the ages of 20 and 69 have noise-induced hearing loss due to a variety of noise types. For children, it is estimated that two to three out of every 1,000 U.S. babies born will have some form of hearing loss (Vohr, O'Shea, & Wright, 2003), and between ages 6 and 17 years an estimated 14.9% of U.S. children will have hearing loss that exceeds 16 dB HL pure tone average (Niskar et al., 1998).

Common approaches for remediating hearing loss include surgical correction (full or partial correction), hearing aids, implantable devices, and alternative communication modalities (e.g., sign language). There have been numerous technological advances over the years, particularly for hearing aids and implantable devices. The use of hearing aids for remediation of hearing loss is the most common, but the adoption rates for hearing aids have long been reported by the industry to be about 20%, with adoption rates as high as 25% (Kochkin, 2009). This means that, at most, only one in four individuals with hearing loss is actually using hearing aids. The prevalence of hearing aid use increases from about 3% to 4% in young adults to about 14% to 30% in older adults (Chien & Lin, 2012; Kochkin, 2009). The U.S. Food and Drug Administration (FDA) has reported, as of December 2012, that there are an estimated 324,200 individuals worldwide with cochlear implants, with about 96,000 of those in the United States, roughly 58,000 adults and 38,000 children. Potential cochlear implant users generally must have a severe to profound hearing loss to qualify for the surgery. What these figures indicate is that there are quite a number of individuals with hearing loss who (1) are not seeking treatment, (2) are unhappy with the performance of hearing aids, or (3) have hearing loss so severe that other strategies have been adopted. The prevalence of hearing loss will only continue to grow, and the need for hearing aids, implantable devices, and other hearing assistive and access technologies will be required to counteract the effects of hearing loss.

What's in This Book?

How do we get access to auditory signals? We offer the information in this book to help you answer that question. We include information on the latest access technologies (e.g., NFC and Bluetooth LE), new uses of older technologies (e.g., induction neck loops with wireless streamers), as well as long-proven technologies (e.g., FM and IR systems) to assist the reader in making the best choices in particular situations for access to the auditory signal. We should be cognizant that not all individuals with hearing loss will benefit from only auditory signal enhancements, and instead, various visual technologies may also be helpful.

This book is laid out in four sections. Foundational information is presented in Section One, including this chapter. Chapter 2 contains information on the federal laws governing access for deaf and hard-of-hearing consumers. Coverage includes one of the first U.S. laws in this arena, the Rehabilitation Act of 1973, through the Twenty-First Century Communications and Video Accessibility Act of 2010. Chapter 3 provides a tutorial on the acoustics of sound as well as the acoustics of various listening environments. Chapter 3 explains the obstacles of reverberation, distance, and background noise and how and why assistive devices are useful for those with hearing loss with each of those barriers to communication. Chapter 4 is an overview of personal amplification such as hearing aids and implantable devices. Features of hearing aids that aid listening in difficult acoustic environments are included (e.g., directional microphones and digital noise reduction). Explanations of how newer technologies, such as wireless communication, have been harnessed for use with personal amplification will help the reader understand the role of personal amplification, both its usefulness and limitations. Rounding out the first section is Chapter 5 on assessing the needs of an individual in terms of assistive technologies for communication. The World Health Organization's health classification model is introduced, along with ideas for implementing that model in audiology, which helps identify an individual's activity limitations and participation restrictions that need to be addressed.

Section Two consists of a group of chapters dedicated to various hearing assistive technologies (HATs). Chapter 6 addresses frequency-modulated (FM) devices and the many uses for them. Chapter 7 contains an explanation of how induction technology works. Also included in this chapter are uses for induction loops, telecoil use in hearing aids, cochlear implants, and bone-anchored implants, and an explanation of how assistive devices can employ telecoils to interface with personal amplification. Chapter 8 explains how an infrared (IR) signal is used to convey sound across a space, as well as various devices available for home and public space use. Chapter 9

introduces the reader to various wireless technologies, some quite familiar such as Wi-Fi and Bluetooth, and others less familiar to many in 2014, such as near-field communication (NFC).

Section Three is dedicated to access through telephones, to television programs and movies, and to alerting and signaling devices for various situations. Chapter 10 covers access to and through various forms of telephones and other telecommunications. Text-based technologies and software and equipment that offer access to the spoken word through speech-to-text and text-to-text translation are presented in Chapter 11. In this chapter, read about access avenues such as closed captioning and an app that provides live speech-to-text translation. Closed captioning can be used both offline, to caption recorded programming, and in real time, for access to live events. Chapter 12 has material about alerting/signaling technologies that can be important for both safety and environmental information. "Mobile phone tips" are included for many of the device types discussed in this chapter, given that mobile phones have become ubiquitous and essential for so many people.

Finally, Section Four contains three informative chapters that did not quite fit in the previous three sections. The reader will find Chapter 13 useful because of the seven case studies, which, together, display a variety of people, settings, and needs for different types of hearing assistive and access technologies. This chapter will help readers "put it all together" as they read about several pieces of equipment used in each case, as well as the specific information about each client which requires unique solutions to prevent or address issues for that person. Chapter 14 will help the reader understand the specialized needs of health care professionals with hearing loss. As an example, listening to heartbeats both on physical examination and when taking blood pressure is a critical skill for many health care professions. Moreover, audiologists with hearing loss working in a hearing-based field will often face challenges related to both speech audiometry and to the care of patients' hearing aids. Hearing loss could compromise these skills, but included in this chapter are assistive technologies and strategies for compensating. To round out and finalize the book, Chapter 15 is a grab bag of relatively new or novel technologies as well as up-and-coming technologies.

References

Agrawal, Y., Platz, E. A., & Niparko, J. K. (2008). Prevalence of hearing loss and differences by demographic characteristics among US adults: Data from the National Health and Nutritional Examination Survey, 1999–2004. *Archives of Internal Medicine, 168*(14), 1522–1530.

Chien, W., & Lin, F. R. (2012). Prevalence of hearing aid use among older adults in the United States. *Archives of Internal Medicine, 172*(3), 292–293.

Kirshman, N. H., & Grandgenett II, R. L. (1997). ADA: The 10 most common disabilities and how to accommodate, *2 LegalBrief L.J. 3*. Retrieved from http://www.LegalBrief.com/kirshman.html

Kochkin, S. (2005). The impact of untreated hearing loss on household income. *Better Hearing Institute.* pp. 1–10. Retrieved from http://www.hearing.org/uploadedFiles/Content/impact_of_untreated_hearing_loss_on_income.pdf

Kochkin, S. (2009). MarkeTrak VIII: 25-year trends in the hearing health market. *Hearing Journal, 16*(11), 12–31.

Le Prell, C. G., Hensley, B. N., Campbell, K. C. M., Hall III, J. W., & Guire, K. (2011). Evidence of hearing loss in a "normally-hearing" college student population. *International Journal of Audiology, 50*(Suppl. 1), S21–S31.

Lin, F. R., Niparko, J. K., & Ferrucci, L. (2011). Hearing loss prevalence in the United States. *Archives of Internal Medicine, 171*(20), 1851–1852.

National Joint Committee for the Communicative Needs of Persons with Severe Disabilities. (1992). Guidelines for meeting the communication needs of persons with severe disabilities. *Asha, 34*(Suppl. 7), 2–3.

Niskar, A. S., Kieszak, S. M., Holmes, A. E., Esteban, E., Rubin, C., & Brody, D. J. (1998). Prevalence of hearing loss among children 6 to 19 years of age: The third National Health and Nutrition Examination Survey. *Journal of the American Medical Association, 279*(14), 1071–1075.

Niskar, A. S., Kieszak, S. M., Holmes, A. E., Esteban, E., Rubin, C., & Brody, D. J. (2001). Estimated prevalence of noise-induced hearing threshold shifts among children 6 to 19 years of age: The Third National Health and Nutrition Examination Survey, 1988–1994, United States. *Pediatrics, 108*(1), 40–43.

U.S. Census Bureau. (2005, June–September). Survey of Income and Program Participation, 2004 Panel, Wave 5.

World Health Organization. (2012). *Millions of people in the world have hearing loss that can be treated or prevented.* World Health Organization. Retrieved from http://www.who.int/pbd/deafness/news/Millionslivewithhearingloss.pdf

Vohr, B. R., O'Shea, M., & Wright, L. L. (2003, August). Longitudinal multicenter follow-up of high-risk infants: Why, who, when, and what to assess. *Seminars in Perinatology, 27*(4), 333–342.

2

Federal Access Laws for Deaf and Hard of Hearing Consumers

Introduction

Most people's natural inclination is to skip or only glance quickly at a chapter on the laws governing disabilities. However, please consider spending some time on this chapter for a few reasons: (1) to become familiar with the primary federal disabilities laws (there are some laws in existence that you may not realize are actual laws); (2) to serve as an advocacy resource for your clients, friends, and family; and (3) to make individuals with hearing loss knowledgeable about their rights under the law. As the saying goes, *knowledge is power* and empowering people with hearing loss to get what

they need in any situation is potent. With the ever-present possibility that the laws presented in this chapter can be amended, we have included in the resources watchdog groups and federal executive branch agencies that stay up-to-date on changes to disability laws and publicize those changes. For example, the U.S. Department of Justice, Civil Rights Division has a webpage entitled *A Guide to Disability Rights Laws* (U.S. DOJ, 2009) that provides up-to-date information on a number of laws and includes the Americans with Disabilities Act (ADA), the Telecommunications Act, the Rehabilitation Act and the Individuals with Disabilities Education Improvement Act, as well as a few others.

In the limited space here, we provide a brief overview of the most relevant portions of the following laws:

- Rehabilitation Act of 1973,
- Individuals with Disabilities Education Improvement Act of 1975,
- Hearing Aid Compatibility Act of 1988,
- Americans with Disabilities Act of 1990, and
- Twenty-First Century Communications and Video Accessibility Act of 2010.

We have chosen to present these laws in chronological order based on when they were first passed. However, each of these, except the Twenty-First Century Communications and Video Accessibility act, has been amended by Congress and/or have had their rules and regulations changed one or more times. We discuss the original law to some degree but also the law and rules and regulations as they stand in 2014, the time of this writing.

Before presenting these legislation summaries, we would like to remind you about the process of law making. Legislative branches of governments (U.S. Congress, state legislatures) pass laws, executive branch agencies (e.g., U.S. Department of Education, Arkansas Department of Education) develop the rules and regulations specifying how the laws are implemented and enforced, and the judicial branch (courts) may decide cases that specify whether the laws and rules and regulations at issue in those cases are constitutional. The point of this reminder is that knowing about a law's rules and regulations as well as relevant court cases is important and, as occurred with the ADA, laws may be amended in response to judicial branch decisions.

The Rehabilitation Act

The Rehabilitation Act of 1973 is largely acknowledged in the United States as the first law in which civil rights were codified for people with disabilities. Many disability rights advocates cite section 504 as the most important component of the Rehabilitation Act. Section 504 prohibits federal government agencies, as well as any employers and organizations who receive federal monies, from discriminating against "qualified individuals with disabilities" with regard to the following activities of the business or organization: service availability, accessibility, delivery, and employment. Individuals cannot be denied the opportunity to participate in or benefit from any federally funded program, service, or benefit and cannot be denied access because of physical barriers.

Who are qualified individuals with disabilities? The Rehabilitation Act included an important definition for this term:

[from Sec. 7] . . . has a physical or mental impairment which substantially limits one or more of such person's major life activities; has a record of such an impairment; or is regarded as having such an impairment . . .

For purposes of employment, *qualified individuals with disabilities* are persons who, with *reasonable accommodation*, can perform the essential functions of the job for which they have applied or have been hired to perform (DHHS, 2006).

The U.S. Department of Health and Human Services' *Fact Sheet* (DHHS, 2006) explains that caring for one's self, walking, seeing, hearing, speaking, breathing, working, performing manual tasks, and learning, are all major life activities. Employers cannot discriminate against individuals with a disability with regard to hiring, promotion, training, or fringe benefits when, with reasonable accommodations provided by the employer, that person can perform the essential functions of a position.

What is a reasonable accommodation? That is a great question, and there is some guidance in the law for employers on this topic. Examples of reasonable accommodations for people with hearing loss would be amplified landline telephones, mobile phones (with texting capability), hearing assistive technology systems (e.g., induction loop in a conference room), and visual and vibrating alerting devices. The types of accommodation(s) will depend on the difficulties an individual experiences in a particular position and company. The law also states that employers must take reasonable steps to accommodate the disability unless those steps cause undue hardship to the employer. "Undue hardship" has generally been interpreted to mean the accommodation is too expensive for that employer to provide. One of the factors that must be considered in deciding whether an accommodation is causing undue hardship is the monetary resources of the company. Thus, an accommodation that causes a 50-employee company undue hardship may be easily provided by a 1,000-employee company.

Individuals With Disabilities Education Improvement Act

This law was originally passed in 1975 as the *Education of All Handicapped Children Act*, Public Law 94-142. There is interesting history that precedes and explains the passage of this federal law. Two lawsuits, *Pennsylvania Association for Retarded Children (PARC) v. Pennsylvania* (PA, 1971) and *Mills v. Board of Education* (DC, 1972), were brought by parents/guardians on behalf of children with disabilities who were either excluded from a free public education or received substandard services for education. In both cases the courts ruled that these children had a right to a free, appropriate public education in the least restrictive environment, citing the equal protection guarantees of the 14th Amendment to the U.S. Constitution. States were then required to comply with the findings of the courts and begin providing free public education to children with disabilities, and by 1975, 30 states had enacted laws to do so (121 Cong. Rec. 19, 487-91 [June 18, 1975]). Costs to states and education districts were quite high. Congress stepped in with this act to send federal dollars to help the states pay for this mandate.

To receive those federal funds, states were required to develop and put policies and programs in place that guaranteed equal access to a free appropriate public education to all children with disabilities. Most of us are familiar with at least some of the provisions of this original legislation, such as (1) the evaluation of children with disabilities and the development of an individualized education program (IEP), with parent input; (2) students with disabilities should be placed in the "least restrictive environment," meaning an environment that allows the maximum interaction with students who have no disabilities; and (3) a due process clause that guarantees an impartial hearing between parents and a school system. Perhaps a lesser known mandate is the directive to provide one free meal each day to children with disabilities. In general, Congress passed this law to meet the following four goals (1) make sure that special education services are available for children with disabilities; (2) guarantee fair and appropriate decisions about those services; (3) establish specific management and auditing requirements for special education; and (4) provide federal funds to help the states educate students with disabilities (Education for All Handicapped Children Act, 1975).

The legislation passed in 1975 received significant overhauls, first in 1989, then in 1997, and most recently in 2004. The 1989 amendments changed the law's name to the *Individuals with Disabilities Education Act* (IDEA) and the 2004 legislation amended the name to the *Individuals with Disabilities Education Improvement Act*. IDEA defines a child with a disability as a "child . . . with an intellectual disability, hearing impairments (including deafness), speech or language impairments, visual impairments (including blindness), serious emotional disturbance, orthopedic impairments, autism, traumatic brain injury, other health impairments or specific learning disabilities" (§602(3)(A)(i), IDEA 2004). Importantly, eligibility for services under IDEA requires the child to fall into one of those diagnostic categories and that the presence of the disability causes that child to require special education and any related services. That is, having a disability in and of itself does not qualify a child to receive special education. Rather, the disability has to be significant enough to cause the child to not be successful without additional or different services at school.

An interesting point is that "assistive technologies" (ATs) are defined as both devices (for example, a hearing aid) and services (any service that directly assists a child in the selection, acquisition, or use of the device, for example, programming the hearing aid). Clarifications of what constitutes assistive technology devices and services are also provided in the statute. We have included the somewhat lengthy but relevant statute text below and draw your attention to the underlined passage (underlining added):

1. Assistive Technology Device
   A. In general: The term "assistive technology device" means any item, piece of equipment, or product system, whether acquired commercially off the

shelf, modified, or customized, that is used to increase, maintain, or improve functional capabilities of a child with a disability.

B. Exception: The term does not include a medical device that is surgically implanted, or the replacement of such device.

2. Assistive Technology Service

The term "assistive technology service" means any service that directly assists a child with a disability in the selection, acquisition, or use of an assistive technology device. Such term includes:

A. the evaluation of the needs of such child, including a functional evaluation of the child in the child's customary environment;

B. purchasing, leasing, or otherwise providing for the acquisition of assistive technology devices by such child;

C. selecting, designing, fitting, customizing, adapting, applying, maintaining, repairing, or replacing assistive technology devices;

D. coordinating and using other therapies, interventions, or services with assistive technology devices, such as those associated with existing education and rehabilitation plans and programs;

E. training or technical assistance for such child, or, where appropriate, the family of such child; and

F. training or technical assistance for professionals (including individuals providing education and rehabilitation services), employers, or other individuals who provide services to, employ, or are otherwise substantially involved in the major life functions of such child. (Sect. 602, IDEA, Pub. L. 108–446, 2004)

Therefore, while devices such as hearing aids, frequency-modulated (FM) boots, Bluetooth streamers, and microphones for teachers are thought of as assistive devices that school districts must provide, implantable medical devices (e.g., cochlear implants and bone-anchored implants) were specifically excluded from the list of items that school districts must purchase. It is still true that cochlear implants and bone-anchored implants are more costly than even the most expensive hearing aids, and school districts have limited resources that must be used for all the children in that district. In exempting implantable devices from the definition of assistive technologies, school districts/public agencies also do not have to pay for services specifically related to implantable devices, such as mapping and maintenance. To audiologists this exclusion probably makes little sense. One explanation for this decision, however, comes from the U.S. Senate Committee on Health, Education, Labor, and Pensions report (S. Rept. No. 108–185, 2003) that mapping and maintenance should not be the responsibility of a school district because they are part of the treatment the family chose and do not have to be performed at the school and during school hours. School districts typically are not required to pay for hearing aid adjustment visits either, which could be viewed as a service similar to mapping. Fortunately, the IDEA (2004) regulations on "related services" do state that even with excluded devices and services, children with implantable (hearing) devices will receive additional, related devices such as FM systems, and related services such as monitoring the function of the device, and speech and language therapy.

The U.S. Department of Education, in writing the rules and regulations for IDEA (2004) have made clear other issues surrounding ATs, for example, who is responsible for purchasing equipment and what processes must occur for every child:

- School districts have to provide ATs at no cost to the family for the school setting and also for the home, if the IEP team decides AT is needed at home to ensure free and appropriate public education (FAPE).
- AT needs will be decided on an individual basis, and AT is required if the child needs that help to access FAPE.
- The IEP has to be clear about what type(s) of AT devices and how much AT services each child will receive.
- Parents are provided procedural protections with an extensive set of procedural safeguards, including the provision of AT to the child. (Assistive Technology Training Online, 2005)

Hearing Aid Compatibility Act

The original Hearing Aid Compatibility Act of 1988 required that wireline (i.e., landline) telephones manufactured within the United States beginning in 1989 had to include hearing aid compatible technology. This mandate included "essential" telephones, defined in the law as "coin-operated telephones, telephones provided for emergency use and other telephones frequently needed for use by persons using . . . hearing aids" [Sect. 3(b)(2)(C)(4)(A)], for example, telephones in hotel rooms and in institutions such as hospitals. In addition to the telephones being mandated to work with hearing aids, the law also required that hearing aids must be designed to work with telephones. Wireless telephones (e.g., mobile phones) and government telephones used to transmit classified information were exempt from this law in the 1988 statute.

This legislation was originally aimed at acoustic and electromagnetic/telecoil technology but not digital technology. Mobile phones, which are actually a type of two-way radio, existed when the law passed; however, the technological needs to make them hearing aid compatible were quite expensive, and Congress, acknowledging that reality, included mobile phones in the exemption. Congress also acknowledged that technology might soon be developed to address the high cost of making mobile phones hearing aid compatible. To accommodate this possibility, Congress granted the Federal Communications Commission (FCC) the power to periodically review the rules and regulations in order to revoke or limit the wireless telephone exemption when hearing aid compatibility became a reasonable requirement for mobile technology. The mobile phone exemption was revisited in 2003. At that point the FCC concluded that the technology available to create compatibility between hearing aids and mobile phones existed and that continuing to exempt mobile phones from the Hearing Aid Compatibility Act had an adverse effect on people with hearing loss. The FCC then established rules for hearing aid compatibility with some (but not all) digital mobile phones.

The FCC has established product standards for hearing aid compatibility with mobile phones. Hearing aids can be compatible with mobile phones through an acoustic coupling, which is measured through the microphone and is rated on a scale of M1–M4, with M1 indicating the weakest coupling and M4 the strongest. Hearing aids can also be compatible through a telecoil, or inductive coupling, and is measured on a scale of T1–T4, with T1 indicating the weakest coupling and T4 the strongest. The FCC rules require a mobile phone to achieve minimum ratings of M3 and T3 on the relevant American National Standards Institute (ANSI, 2007 or ANSI, 2011) standard to be considered hearing aid compliant and to carry those designations on the packaging or in the product manual (FCC, 2012).

Some handset manufacturers offer devices that are capable of using wireless technologies, for example, Wi-Fi and Bluetooth. As of 2014, ANSI does not have product standards for this type of handset to be compliant with hearing aids. This is not to say that those handsets will not work with hearing aids, but there is not a specified, standardized way to test those connections at present.

The Americans With Disabilities Act

The Americans with Disabilities Act (ADA), first passed in 1990 and amended in 2008, is perhaps the most well-known U.S. law regarding nondiscrimination of individuals with disabilities. Passage of the ADA significantly strengthened U.S. law with regard to persons with disabilities, building on the Rehabilitation Act of 1973, the Individuals with Disabilities Education Improvement Act of 1975, and their amendments.

The ADA of 1990 has five titles or sections: Title I—Employment, Title II—Public Services, Title III—Public Accommodations and Services Operated by Private Entities, Title IV—Telecommunications, and Title V—Miscellaneous Provisions. Title I states that employers with 15 or more employees cannot discriminate against individuals with disabilities in application procedures, hiring, promotion, firing, compensation, or training opportunities. Title I excludes the U.S. Government, Indian tribes, and private membership clubs. Covered individuals are those with a disability who can perform the essential functions of the job either with or without reasonable accommodation (ADA, 2008). Employers decide what functions are essential for each position and must provide "reasonable accommodation" that does not cause "undue hardship" to the employer. As with the Rehabilitation Act, the phrases "reasonable accommodation" and "undue hardship" warrant explanation. The Department of Health and Human Services explains that "reasonable accommodation means an employer is required to take reasonable steps to accommodate your disability unless it would cause the employer undue hardship." (DHHS Fact Sheet, p. 1). Reasonable accommodation may include changing existing facilities or restructuring jobs, work schedules, or equipment, in order for the individual with a disability to perform the job. Undue hardship refers to an action causing significant difficulty or expense for the employer, and several factors to consider are included, for example, the nature and cost of the accommodation and the available financial resources of the employer. Furthermore, employers cannot ask directly about a disability of a person applying for a job but can ask about that person's ability to perform particular job functions.

Title II mandates that no state and local governments, their departments and agencies, nor commuter authorities (e.g., the Chicago Transit Authority) can discriminate against someone with a disability regarding access to and participation in programs and services the agency provides. One of the most visible results of this title was the addition of wheelchair lifts on public conveyances, for example, city buses, and local government programs that provide transportation to appointments for people with disabilities.

For individuals with hearing loss this title resulted in the addition of teletypewriter/telecommunication devices for the deaf (TTY/TDD) to access government offices and assistive device technology availability in public venues such as hotels and concert halls.

Title III addresses discrimination toward those with disabilities in "public accommodations and services operated by private entities." In plain language, many business types are identified as "public accommodation" and must adhere to the provisions of this title. Examples of these business types include hotels, restaurants, theaters, stadiums, convention centers, depots, stores, galleries, social service centers, and gyms. Basically, all businesses except private clubs and religious organizations are covered. For covered businesses, Title III mandates that the experiences provided by these businesses cannot be denied to those with disabilities, cannot be separate from, and must equal the experiences of those with no disabilities. The statute further states that businesses must make reasonable modifications to accommodate individuals with disabilities.

Title IV, telecommunications, actually amended a portion of the Communications Act of 1934. Common carriers in inter- and intrastate communication by wire or radio (note that wireless was not included in the original law) are covered in this title. One of the primary mandates of Title IV is the establishment of telecommunication relay services for people in the United States with hearing and/or speech impairments. The interstate version of this service is paid for by customers of the various communication companies, typically a 50¢ charge on one's bill. States are also allowed to set up a relay service for in-state use. One further mandate is that public service announcements for television produced or funded by the federal government must have closed captioning and that television stations airing those announcements must broadcast the closed captioning.

Title V is a miscellany addressing various aspects and consequences of the ADA. For example, Title V states that individuals with disabilities are not required to accept accommodations or services; states can be sued for not following the ADA; people who oppose practices that the ADA made unlawful cannot be retaliated against; and, anyone who takes advantage of this law for themselves or encourages others to do so cannot be coerced or intimidated because of that stand. The U.S. Senate and House of Representatives specifically included themselves as subject to the ADA in employment and physical access issues. Importantly, enforcement procedures are included in the ADA and the rules and regulations of the various agencies overseeing the various parts of the law's implementation contain information for consumers on how to lodge complaints.

Why Congress Amended the ADA

When an individual lodges a complaint or lawsuit against any entity under the ADA, that individual must first demonstrate that she or he has a disability. In other words, they must qualify as having a disability to be covered under the law. In the original legislation, "disability" was defined with the following three phrases: (1) a physical or mental impairment that substantially limits one or more of the major life activities of such individual, (2) a record of such an impairment, or (3) being regarded as having such an impairment. There was no additional or specific language that explained when an individual should be considered to have a disability and no further explanation of major life activities. The definition of disability did not change in the 2008 version of the ADA; however, Congress added the following language so that there would be no doubt that Congress intended more people with more conditions be covered under the ADA rather than fewer:

[from Sect. 3(2)(A)] . . . major life activities include, but are not limited to, caring for oneself, performing manual tasks, seeing, hearing, eating, sleeping, walking, standing, lifting, bending, speaking, breathing, learning, reading, concentrating, thinking, communicating, and working.

. . . a major life activity also includes the operation of a major bodily function, including but not limited to, functions of the immune system, normal cell growth, digestive, bowel, bladder, neurological, brain, respiratory, circulatory, endocrine, and reproductive functions.

Congress added additional language to give further clarity:

[from Sect. 4]

C. An impairment that substantially limits one major life activity need not limit other major life activities in order to be considered a disability.

D. An impairment that is episodic or in remission is a disability if it would substantially limit a major life activity when active.

E. The determination of whether an impairment substantially limits a major life activity shall be made without regard to the ameliorative effects of mitigating measures such as

  I. medication, medical supplies, equipment, or appliances, low-vision devices (which do not include ordinary eyeglasses or contact lenses), prosthetics including limbs and devices, hearing aids and cochlear implants or other implantable hearing devices, mobility devices, or oxygen therapy equipment and supplies;

  II. use of assistive technology;

  III. reasonable accommodations or auxiliary aids or services; or

  IV. learned behavioral or adaptive neurological modifications.

In the amended ADA legislation of 2008, Congressional explanations for the amendments indicate that when the ADA was passed in 1990 Congress expected that courts would interpret "disability" as they had previously interpreted "handicapped individual" under the Rehabilitation Act of 1973. However, that definition was not applied and in at least two court cases, *Sutton v. United Air Lines, Inc.* U.S. 471 (1999) and *Toyota Motor Manufacturing, Kentucky, Inc. v. Williams*, 534 U.S. 184 (2002), the courts narrowed the broad protection Congress had intended. Congress then clarified the law, giving less room for interpretation by the courts of what was meant by "disability."

In *Sutton v. United Air Lines, Inc.* U.S. 471 (1999) and accompanying cases, the U.S. Supreme Court held that a business or government agency could consider devices and medication that might lessen the impact of a person's health condition before deciding whether that person has a disability. In the second case, *Toyota v. Williams* (2002), the U.S. Supreme Court found that to have a disability, a person had to show that everyday tasks "of central importance to most people's daily lives" were affected permanently, and not only job-specific tasks. In essence, the Supreme Court's ruling required individuals to have a higher level of disability than Congress intended in order to be covered by the ADA. In its response legislation, the 2008 ADA Amendments Act (ADAAA), Congress mentioned these two cases specifically saying that the Supreme Court and the Equal Employment Opportunity Commission had limited protection of the law more than Congress had intended. Thus, the ADAAA specifically states that the decision on whether a person has a disability must be based on that person's health condition(s) without considering any devices or medications she/he might use and included a definition for the term *disability* [see the quote Sect. 3(2)(A) above], which removed the opportunity for the courts' interpretation.

Twenty-First Century Communications and Video Accessibility Act

The Twenty-First Century Communications and Video Accessibility Act of 2010 (CVAA) was passed to ensure that new types/technologies of communication and communication devices are made accessible to people who have hearing loss. Companies that distribute video and television broadcasts must provide closed captioning to assist deaf and hard of hearing viewers. Videos developed strictly for the Internet do not have to have closed captioning nor do videos embedded into a website that require a third-party video player, such as JavaScript (SSB Bart Group, 2013). Internet content that is generated by consumers (many of the videos on YouTube) is not required to have captioning. Presenting these ideas in more detail, Title I of the law deals with communications access and "advanced communication services," defined as (a) interconnected voice over Internet protocol (VoIP); (b) noninterconnected VoIP; (c) electronic messaging, for example, text message, e-mail, and instant messaging; and (d) interoperable video conferencing. Relevant mandates from Title I are as follows:

- Advanced communications services and products must be accessible to individuals with disabilities.
- Hearing aids and all advanced communications services must be compatible.

- The FCC must have a clearinghouse on accessible communications services and equipment (http://ach.fcc.gov/) .
- The FCC is required to respond to and close consumer complaints within 180 days; complaints on accessibility may be lodged at http://www.fcc.gov/complaints.
- Up to $10 million per year is sent from the Interstate Telecommunications Relay Service Fund for specialized equipment to be distributed to low-income individuals who are deaf-blind.
- Authorizes FCC action to ensure that persons with disabilities will have reliable and interoperable access *to next-generation 9-1-1* services (Twenty-First Century Communications and Video Accessibility Act of 2010).

Title II covers video programming. Some of this title's requirements are listed below:

- Television programs (except live programs) with closed captioning must also be closed captioned if distributed on the Internet, but programs shown only on the Internet using third-party software such as JavaScript are not covered.
- Any device with a screen smaller than 13″ (e.g., portable TVs, laptops, tablets, mobile phones) that can display a television

program must be able to display closed captions *if technically feasible and achievable as determined by the FCC* (italics added).

- Devices with screens smaller than 13″ must be capable of sending video descriptions and emergency information for individuals who are blind or visually impaired, *if technically feasible and achievable as determined by the FCC* (italics added).
- Remote control devices must be accessible and must have a mechanism (e.g., button, key, icon) that activates the closed captioning and video description.

Summary

Over the previous four decades, the U.S. Government has passed and implemented many important pieces of legislation to ensure that individuals with physical and/or mental disabilities are included in all aspects of society. It is important that we, as professionals who work with people who have hearing loss, remain up-to-date on current laws, when and how they are amended, and understand the impact of those changes for our clients.

References

Accessibility Management Platform. (2013). *CVAA Advanced Communica-tion Services–AMP.* SSB Bart Group. Retrieved from https://www.ssbbart group.com/reference/index.php/CVAA_Advanced_Communication _Services

ADA Amendments Act of 2008, Pub. L. 110-325, codified as amended at 42 USCA § 12101 note. Retrieved from http://www.eeoc.gov/laws/statutes/adaaa.cfm

American National Standards Institute. (2007, 2011). *C63.19—Methods of measurement of compatibility between wireless communications devices and hearing aids.* doi:10.1109/IEEESTD .2011.5782919

Americans with Disabilities Act of 1990, Pub. L. 101-336, 104 Stat. 327. (1990). Retrieved from http://www.gpo.gov/fdsys/pkg/STATUTE-104/pdf/STAT-UTE-104-Pg327.pdf

Assistive Technology Training Online Project. (2005). *AT & IDEA.* University of Buffalo School of Public Health and Health Professions. Retrieved from http://atto.buffalo.edu/registered/ATBasics/Foundation/intro/introAT idea.php

Consumer and Governmental Affairs Bureau, Federal Communication Commission. (n.d.). *21st Century communications and video accessibility act (VCAA).* (FCC Consumer Facts). Retrieved from http://transition.fcc.gov/cgb/consumerfacts/CVAA-access-act .pdf

Consumer and Governmental Affairs Bureau, Federal Communication Commission. (2012). *Hearing aid compatibility for wireless telephones.* (FCC Consumer Facts). Retrieved from http://

transition.fcc.gov/cgb/consumerfacts/hac_wireless.pdf

Disability Rights Section, Civil Rights Division, U.S. Department of Justice. (2009). *A guide to disability rights laws.* Retrieved from http://www.ada.gov/cguide.htm#anchor62335

Hearing Aid Compatibility Act of 1988, Pub. L. 100-394, 102 Stat. 976, codified as amended at 47 U.S.C. §§ 609 note. Retrieved from http://transition.fcc.gov/Bureaus/OSEC/library/legislative_histories/1337.pdf

Individuals with Disabilities Education Act of 1989, Pub. L. 91–230, Title VI, as added Pub. L. 108–446, Title I, § 101, Dec. 3, 2004, 118 Stat. 2647 codified as amended at 20 U.S.C. $1400 et seq.

Kochkin, S. (2010). The efficacy of hearing aids in achieving compensation equity in the workplace, *The Hearing Journal, 63*(10), 19–28.

Office for Civil Rights, U.S. Department of Health and Human Services. (2006). *Your Rights Under Section 504 of the Rehabilitation Act.* Retrieved from http://www.hhs.gov/ocr/civilrights/resources/factsheets/504.pdf

Rehabilitation Act of 1973, Pub. L. 93–112, 87 Stat. 355, codified as amended at 29 U.S.C. §701 et seq. Retrieved from http://www.usbr.gov/cro/pdfsplus/rehabact.pdf

Twenty-First Century Communications and Video Accessibility Act of 2010, Pub. L. 111–260, 124 Stat. 2751, codified as amended at 47 U.S.C. §609 note. Retrieved from http://www.gpo.gov/fdsys/pkg/PLAW-111publ260/pdf/PLAW-111publ260.pdf

United States Senate Committee on Health, Education, Labor, and Pensions. (2003). Individuals with Disabilities Education Act Report 108-185.

3

Acoustic Issues in a Variety of Listening Environments

Review of Acoustics

With or without hearing loss, listening and communicating in different environments can be challenging. Noise and speech are not typically a good combination when communicating via the spoken word. Too often we find ourselves in difficult listening situations with no means of improving the situation, except to remove ourselves from that environment. The better we understand acoustics, the better we can improve those listening situations. Before we can appreciate the acoustic factors associated with listening situations, we need to be familiar with basic acoustics and the concept of sound propagation. This chapter introduces or reviews some of the concepts of acoustics and how sound interacts with its environment.

Before sound is present in an environment, the particles in the air tend to move in a random manner, known as *Brownian motion*. Sound can be thought of as the transfer of energy though an elastic medium. The medium can be anything that can carry this energy from one location to another. For the purposes of this book, we think of air, mostly, as the medium through which sound travels. Further, we may think of sound as vibrations moving through the air and originating from a vibrating object or sound source. These vibrations superimpose their patterns of motion onto those particles that are moving according to Brownian motion. The patterns of motion follow a pattern of greater density, called condensation, and of lesser density, called rarefaction. Notice in Figure 3–1, when energy is added to the tuning fork, it is set into vibration and causes the air particles nearby to vibrate also.

This results in a dynamic partnership between the object's (or medium's) inertial force and its elastic force. The inertial force is influenced by an object's mass. Because density is defined as mass per unit volume, the object's mass affects its inertial properties. Isaac Newton explained this with the first of his three laws of motion. Basically, an object in motion (or at rest) will remain in motion (or at rest) until it is acted upon by an

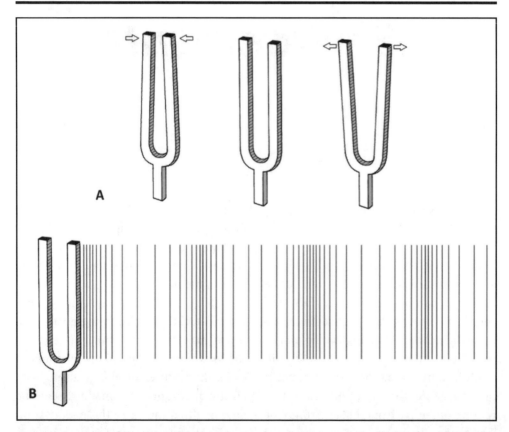

Figure 3–1. When energy is applied to an object having mass and elasticity, the object will vibrate. **A.** After applying energy by striking, the tuning fork vibrates by changing shape, depending on its mass and elasticity. **B.** The tuning fork transfers the vibration to the surrounding air particles in waves of condensation and rarefaction.

external force. The mass of the object will influence how much force is required to affect its motion (or rest). We know that a great deal of force is needed to make a resting object with great mass, like a freight train, begin to roll. When that train is rolling, we know that we will need a lot of force to bring it to a stop. A child's ball will need much less force to cause it to roll or to stop it from rolling. When comparing the train with the ball, it is easy to see that mass plays a role in inertia. The elastic force of an object is its tendency to return to its original shape. When we stretch a rubber band, we are distorting its shape. When we release it, the rubber band's tendency to return to its original shape is known as elasticity. Sometimes elasticity is referred to as the stiffness of an object. We can think about the allegorical comparison between the rigid oak tree and the limber willow tree and conclude that both trees are elastic but differ in the degree of elasticity. Although we may not think of solid objects, like glass, tile, wood, and metal as being elastic, we can appreciate that they can be subtly distorted before they return back to their original shape.

With a vibrating object, amplitude refers to the amount of displacement or distortion in shape as the object vacillates between the influence of inertia and elasticity. In acoustics, amplitude is reflected by the degree of pressure change between the condensation phase and the rarefaction phase, the pattern which is superimposed on the air particles. The unit of measure for this change in amplitude, or the intensity of a sound is the decibel for sound pressure level (dB SPL). The intensity unit, *dB SPL*, is commonly used with hearing aids, hearing assistive and access technology, and noise. The term *cycle* can be thought of as a complete series of occurrences (e.g., the transition from condensation to rarefaction and back to condensation). The term *period* tells us the time that it takes to complete one full cycle, while *wavelength* (λ) tells us the distance required to complete a cycle. Figure 3–2 illustrates the comparison between the tuning fork vibrating, amplitude, period, and wavelength.

Period and wavelength both share an inverse, proportional relationship with frequency. Frequency, in hertz (Hz), can be thought of as the number of cycles completed in 1 second. As wavelength and period increase in magnitude, frequency will decrease proportionally, or with the same magnitude. As Figure 3–3 shows, an example of an inversely proportional relationship is that of a lever, in which the two ends move the same distance, but in opposite directions.

While vibrations can travel through and originate from any object with mass and elasticity, including material such as water and steel, among others; the speed at which sound travels thorough an object or a medium varies based on the object's inertial (i.e., mass) and elastic properties. To illustrate this, we can compare the approximate speed of sound traveling through air (350 m/s), through water (1,500 m/s), and through steel (5,000 m/s). Sound travels faster through solid objects than through air. Even though solid objects are denser than air, they hold much greater elastic properties than air.

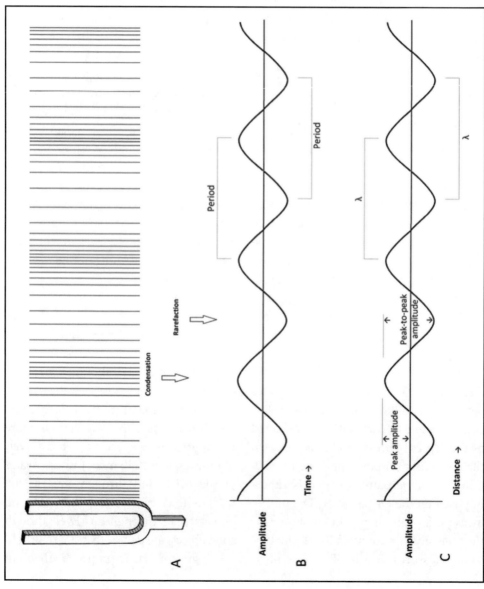

Figure 3–2. A. The tuning fork transfers the vibration to the surrounding air particles in waves of rarefaction and condensation. **B.** When we graph the changes in pressure as a function of time, we see condensation, positive pressure, represented as positive peaks. Rarefaction, negative pressure, is represented by troughs or valleys. Notice that period is the length of time for the sound to complete one full cycle. **C.** When we graph the changes in pressure as a function of distance, we again see condensation represented as positive peaks and rarefaction represented as troughs or valleys. Notice that wavelength is the distance that the sound to travels during one full cycle.

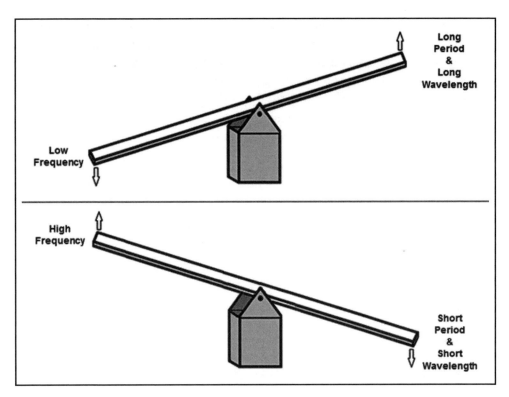

Figure 3–3. An inversely proportional relationship. The two ends of the fulcrum move the same amount, but in opposite directions. This same, inversely proportional relationship exists between frequency and wavelength, and frequency and period.

The speed of sound (c) is equal to the sound's wavelength (λ) multiplied by its frequency (f). This equation can be used to determine the wavelength of a sound with all of its energy at one frequency, known as a pure tone, if we know that frequency:

$$c = \lambda \times f$$

$$\lambda = c \div f$$

$$f = c \div \lambda$$

To calculate the wavelength for a 1000 Hz tone, knowing the speed of sound is 350 m/s, we plug in this information into the appropriate equation and calculate the wavelength:

$$\lambda = c \div f$$

$$\lambda = 350 \text{ m/s} \div 1000 \text{ Hz}$$

$$\lambda = 0.35 \text{ m (or 35 cm)}$$

Phase, or the phase angle, represents the particular point in the cycle. We can think of the amplitude of a tone at a particular point in time, or phase, in the same way we think of observing a full moon on a particular evening. The amplitude of the tone will vary at different phases of its cycle much like the amount of light reflected off the moon varies at different phases of its cycle. Phase is not something that we notice when we are listening to a pure tone. However, we do notice when two or more tones of different phases interact with each other. These interactions result in variations of the sound as illustrated in Figure 3–4. Panel B, with the two tones completely out-of-phase results in cancellation of the tones. The condensation phase of one tone, positive pressure, is countered by the rarefaction

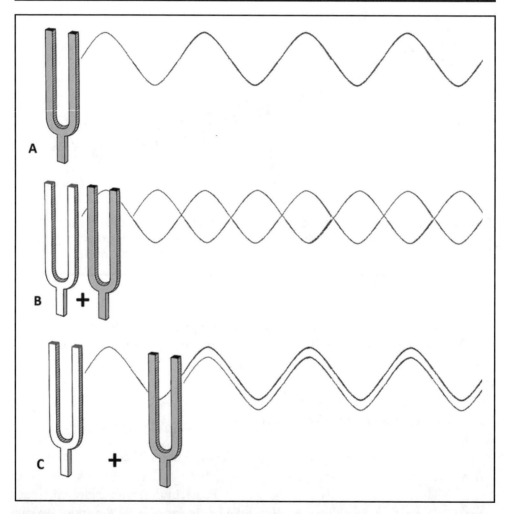

Figure 3–4. A. A single tuning fork transmitting vibrations. **B.** Two tuning forks transmitting vibrations that are 180° out-of-phase. Each vibration will cancel the other out, resulting in no vibration. **C.** Two tuning forks transmitting vibrations that are in-phase. Each vibration will add to the other, resulting in a doubling of amplitude.

phase, negative pressure, of the other tone. The resulting amplitude will be zero. However, in Panel C, the two pure tones are in-phase with each other. The condensation phase of one tone is enhanced by the condensation phase of the other tone; conversely, the rarefaction phase of one tone is enhanced by the rarefaction phase of the other tone. The resulting amplitude will be doubled.

Listening Environments

Why is a review of basic acoustics necessary? When we think about listening in any environment, we need to understand how sound behaves and interacts with the environment before we can successfully address the challenges related to understanding speech in that environment. Every listening situation will be affected by the type, frequency, and level of the signal, the position of the speaker, the position of the listener, the level of the noise present, the distance between the listener and the speaker, and the reverberation of the room.

Speech

When listening to speech, we need to consider the factors associated with acoustics of speech. This includes how the acoustics of that sound contribute to the power and the intelligibility of the speech sound. For the purposes of this book, only a brief description of speech acoustics is provided. More detailed descriptions of the acoustics of speech are provided by Kent and Read (1992) and Lass (1996). Because vowels are produced with a constant flow of air, they typically have more energy than consonants. Figure 3–5 illustrates the typical frequency and intensity of a few speech sounds on an audiogram. In addition, vowels are characterized as having most of their energy in low frequencies. For example, the first formant for vowels (i.e., the frequency regions where much, if not most, of the energy is located) range from about 300 to 800 Hz (Kent & Read, 1992). Figure 3–6 illustrates how the energy can be spread across frequencies, as indicated by relative amplitude, for a vowel. Primarily, a listener can identify the vowel by the relationship between its formants (e.g., energy peaks) and the duration of the vowel. The identification of consonants is more complex, as there is a wide variety of consonants and multiple acoustic cues associated with each consonant sound. Generally speaking, identification of consonants includes perceiving very small changes in intensity (intensity cues), frequency (spectral cues), time (temporal cues), or any combination of these. As compared to vowels, consonants do not have as much energy and are identified more by their second and third formant energy, which typically range from 1000 to 3000 Hz (Kent & Read, 1992). It is for these and other reasons, not included, that vowels contribute more to the power of the speech signal than consonants. Consonants, however, contribute more than vowels to the intelligibility of the speech signal. Individuals

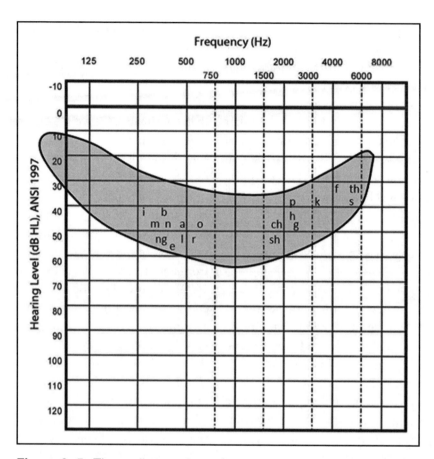

Figure 3–5. The audiogram is an instrument used to graph hearing sensitivity. Speech sounds can be graphed to provide additional applicable information related to hearing sensitivity. The shaded area is often referred to as the "Speech Banana."

with hearing loss in the high frequencies are likely to have difficulty understanding speech because they have trouble hearing consonants due to the frequency region of the hearing loss and because these consonants contribute more to the intelligibility of the speech signal. This is why these individuals may comment that they hear people speak, but that it appears that the speakers mumble or "don't speak clearly."

Distance

When thinking about the effect of distance on sound energy, you have likely noticed that a sound becomes louder if we move closer to the source and softer if we move farther from it. These changes in our perception of loudness are based on the principle that sound spreads or distributes itself over larger and larger

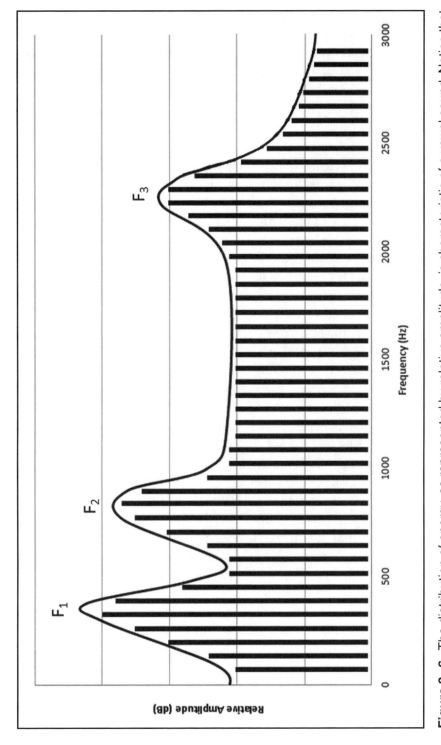

Figure 3–6. The distribution of energy, as represented by relative amplitude, is characteristic of a vowel sound. Notice that most of the energy is located in the first couple of formants (F_1, F_2). The relationship between the formants provides listeners with a cue to distinguish one vowel from another.

areas as it travels farther from the source. This phenomenon is known as the *Inverse Square Law*. Every time that we double our distance, or move twice as far away from the sound, the intensity of the sound will decrease by 6 dB. Conversely, the intensity of the sound will increase by 6 dB if we move closer, by half the distance, to the source of the sound. A change of 6 dB is noticeable, if not significant, in our ability to understand what has been said. For reference, if a tone is increased by 10 dB, the sound will be perceived to be twice as loud. Figures 3–7 and 3–8 help demonstrate how distance can play a role in our ability to understand speech in these two listening environments. The intensity of the speaker's voices will drop by 6 dB SPL each time the distance from that speaker is doubled. If the noise level across the room in Figure 3–6 were 55 dB SPL and those on the front row received the speech signal at 65 dB SPL, they would benefit from a signal being 10 dB greater than the noise level (i.e., a +10 dB signal-to-noise ratio). But, for those twice the distance from the speaker than those in the front row, the speech signal has dropped 6 dB to 59 dB SPL. The result is that those on the second row would receive a speech signal only 4 dB greater than the noise level. If we double that distance, for those sitting on the fourth row of seats, the intensity of the speech signal is 53 dB SPL, while the noise level remains at 55 dB SPL. Those in Figure 3–6 on the fourth row would have to listen to speech embedded in noise (i.e., the noise is 2 dB greater than the speech signal). Figure 3–7 also illustrates the Inverse Square Law within

a conference room. Again, the doubling of distance results in the reduction of the signal by 6 dB. With noise present, those sitting farthest away from the speaker will be hindered by the drop in intensity as the speech signal travels to reach them.

The Inverse Square Law is not the only factor affecting the intensity of the signal. The sound of the speaker's voice will interact with the surrounding surfaces, like light being reflected off a mirror. Sound will be reflected off an object, like a wall (Figure 3–9A). It can also be transmitted through the object (Figure 3–9B). Some of the sound will be absorbed by the object. The remaining sound will be diffracted, or splintered into multiple directions, off the object. Note that the listening environments illustrated in Figures 3–7 and 3–8 indicate how the intensity of the sound decreases as a function of distance alone, but they do not illustrate any other effects of the sound interacting with its surroundings.

Reverberation

Sound travels in all directions away from the source of the sound. More energy may be focused in one direction than others, but sound spreads like a growing sphere. As the sound travels in multiple directions, it will interact with the environment. How the sound travels depends on the size, shape, and materials in the environment. Sound can and will be reflected, transmitted, absorbed, and diffracted off of the surfaces of objects in an environment. These surfaces include,

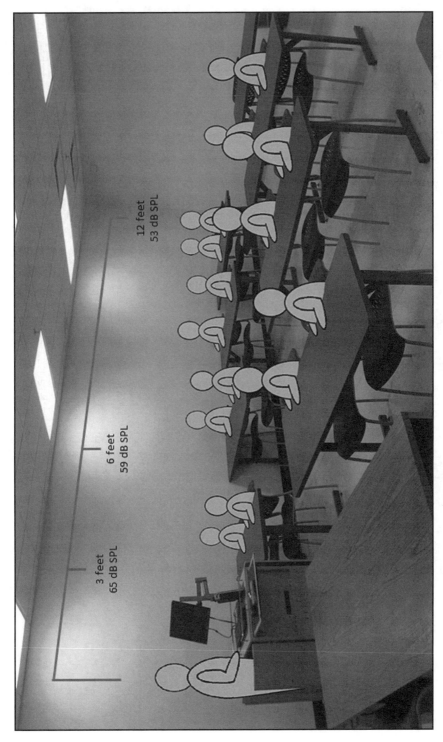

Figure 3–7. The Inverse Square Law illustrated in a classroom environment. Notice that each doubling of distance between the student and the teacher results in a 6 dB drop in intensity.

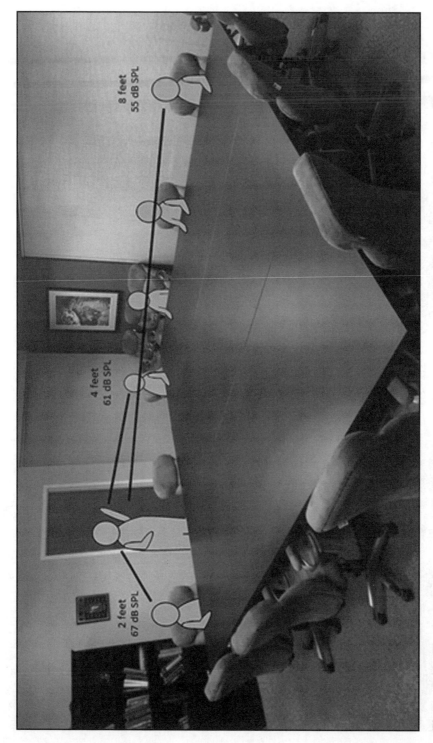

Figure 3–8. The Inverse Square Law illustrated in a conference room. As in Figure 3–5, each doubling of distance between the speaker and the attendees results in a 6 dB drop in intensity.

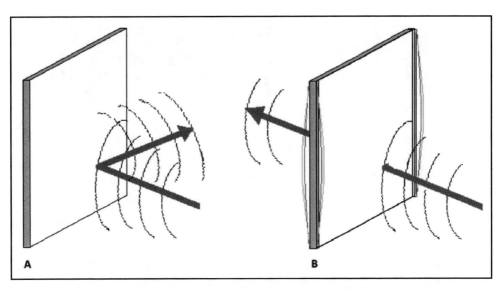

Figure 3–9. How sound is interacting with a wall in a couple of different ways. **A.** The sound energy is reflected off of the wall. **B.** The sound energy is transmitted through the wall.

but are not limited to, walls, ceilings, floors, tables, chairs, people, and furniture. A common situation, incidentally hearing someone through a wall from another room, is shown in Figure 3–10. The sound energy is being transmitted via the wall. Not illustrated in Figure 3–10 is the energy that has been diffracted or absorbed by the wall.

We may think of a reflected sound as an echo. In acoustics, the term used to describe the reflected sound is reverberation. Figure 3–11 illustrates just a few of the pathways through which the sound of the speaker's voice will travel en route to the listener. As time progresses, the sound in the room will continue to be reflected off every object and surface until there is not enough energy for it to continue.

Figure 3–12 illustrates the characteristic decay of sound with and without reverberation. The sound will remain for a longer period of time in a reverberant room. Reverberation can be both good and bad. Some reverberation provides the listener with a richer sound, much like singing in the shower. Too much reverberation can interfere with understanding speech, much like listening to a public address system at a stadium or arena where to speech overlaps itself. Comparatively, more reverberation is preferred in structures designed for listening to live music (e.g., concert halls, cathedrals, etc.) than listening to speech (e.g., classrooms, boardrooms, etc.).

How much sound is reflected off a surface will depend on the surface. Heavy,

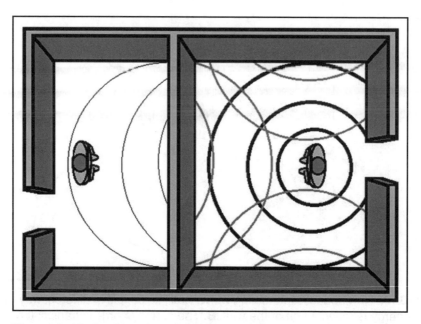

Figure 3–10. Looking down into two rooms where sound is transmitted through a wall. The speaker in one room (right) is heard by someone in the adjacent room (left). The speaker's voice will likely sound muffled as the absorption capabilities of a wall will often absorb more high-frequency components of the speech than the low-frequency components.

thick walls allow for less energy to be transmitted from one room to another, compared to thinner walls, doors, and windows. This difference is because the sound energy causes objects (i.e., walls, doors, windows, etc.) to vibrate. These objects, like air, also have mass and elasticity. This is why we may hear a speaker from a different room.

Different building materials vary in both mass and elasticity, and how sound interacts with different building materials will also differ. To provide more insight into the relationship between building materials and sound, absorption coeffi-cients are used. Absorption coefficients provide us with a metric to use in comparing how sound interacts with different materials. These coefficients indicate the ratio between how much sound energy is reflected versus unreflected from a surface of a particular building material. From Table 3–1, we can see the different absorption coefficients for different materials. The table also shows how different objects interact with sound at different frequencies.

Reverberation time is defined as the amount of time required for the intensity of a sound to decrease by 60 dB, denoted

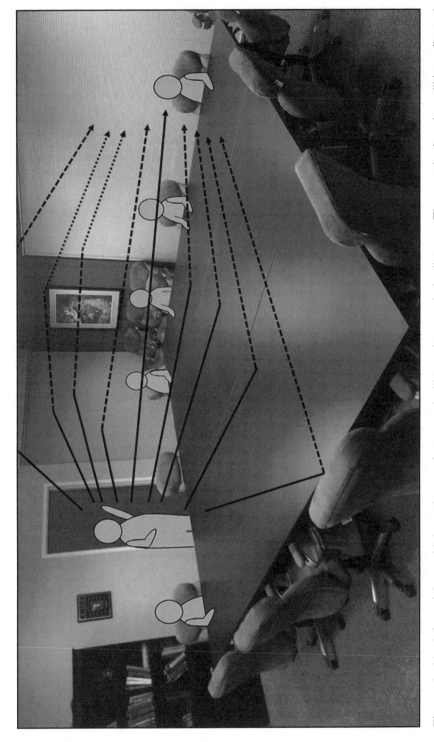

Figure 3–11. A few of the multiple pathways that sound will travel to reach the listener. The speaker's voice will be reflected off the objects in the room until it loses energy to travel any farther. The listener, at a distance, may notice greater difficulty understanding the speaker as the time required to travel each path is different from other paths.

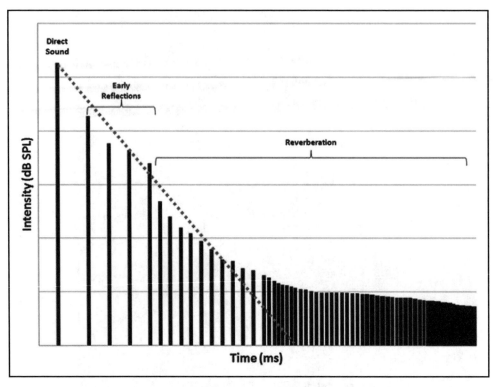

Figure 3–12. The manner in which the intensity of a sound decreases at a constant rate over time and how the intensity of that same sound may be sustained for a longer time due to reverberation.

by RT_{60}. The graph in Figure 3–13 displays the average RT_{60} for three rooms: a large classroom, a small classroom, and a small conference room at 500; 1000; and 2000 Hz. All rooms have 9′ ceilings; but both the small classroom (23′ × 19′) and large classroom (26′ × 37′) have tile floors, hard surfaced tables and chairs, painted drywall (e.g., sheetrock or gypsum), and acoustic ceiling tile. The conference room is 23′ × 25′, approximately the same size as the small classroom, but has a carpeted floor, chairs with cloth and cushion coverings, art on the drywall, some window

treatments (blinds), and acoustic ceiling tile. Notice the difference in RT_{60} for the three rooms in Figure 3–13, especially the differences between the small classroom and the conference room.

RT_{60} values allow us to determine critical distance, the distance away from the sound source where the amount of reverberant or reflected sound equals the amount of direct sound. For any position in the room beyond this critical distance, the listener is exposed to more energy from sounds reflected off of surfaces than from the sound coming directly from the

Table 3–1. Surface Types With Their Corresponding Sound Absorption Coefficients for the Octave Frequencies Between 125 and 4000 Hz

Location	Material	125 Hz	250 Hz	500 Hz	1000 Hz	2000 Hz	4000 Hz
Ceiling	Acoustic ceiling tiles	0.7	0.66	0.72	0.92	0.88	0.75
Floor	Carpet on foam	0.08	0.24	0.57	0.69	0.71	0.73
Wall	Thick curtains	0.14	0.35	0.55	0.72	0.7	0.65
Floor	Carpet on concrete	0.02	0.06	0.14	0.37	0.6	0.65
Wall	Glass window	0.35	0.25	0.18	0.12	0.07	0.04
Wall/ceiling	Wood	0.28	0.22	0.17	0.09	0.1	0.11
Wall	Thin curtains	0.03	0.04	0.11	0.17	0.24	0.35
Wall/ceiling	Sheetrock	0.29	0.1	0.05	0.04	0.07	0.09
Floor	Wood on joists	0.15	0.11	0.1	0.07	0.06	0.07
Ceiling	Wood	0.15	0.11	0.1	0.07	0.06	0.07
Wall	Painted concrete block	0.1	0.05	0.06	0.07	0.09	0.08
Wall/ceiling	Plaster	0.013	0.015	0.02	0.03	0.04	0.05
Wall	Painted brick	0.01	0.01	0.02	0.02	0.02	0.03
Floor	Concrete or tile	0.01	0.01	0.015	0.02	0.02	0.02
Wall	Marble/tile	0.01	0.01	0.01	0.01	0.02	0.02

source. Table 3–2 provides estimated critical distances.

For us as listeners, the critical distance is more of a factor for speech sounds than environmental sounds (i.e., smoke alarm, telephone ringing, etc.). For a complex signal such as speech, the critical distance indicates the distance from a speaker where timing delays begin to become a factor in the ability to understand speech. Just past the critical distance may not cause us much difficulty. It may even provide a rich quality to the speaker's voice, such as singing in the shower.

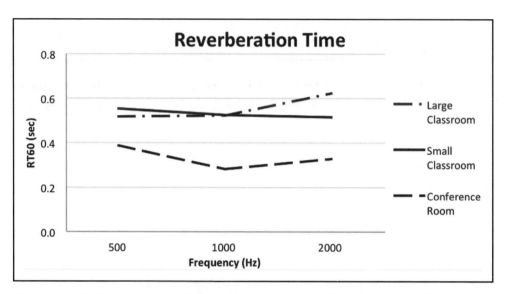

Figure 3–13. Reverberation time in three rooms of different sizes. The average RT_{60} of three rooms is graphed as a function of frequency, specifically 500, 1000, and 2000 Hz.

Table 3–2. Estimated Critical Distances Based on Room Size and Reverberation Time

Room Volume (cubic ft.)	Reverberation Time (seconds)							
	0.3	0.4	0.5	0.6	0.7	0.8	0.9	1.0
2,000	5.2	4.5	4.0	3.7	3.4	3.2	3.0	2.8
4,000	7.3	6.3	5.7	5.2	4.8	4.5	4.2	4.0
6,000	8.9	7.7	6.9	6.9	5.9	5.5	5.2	4.9
8,000	10.3	8.9	8.0	8.0	6.8	6.3	6.0	5.7
10,000	11.5	10.0	8.9	8.9	7.6	7.1	6.7	6.3
12,000	12.6	11.0	9.8	9.8	8.3	7.7	7.3	6.9
14,000	13.7	11.8	10.6	10.6	9.7	8.4	7.9	7.5
16,000	14.6	12.6	11.3	11.3	10.3	8.9	8.4	8.0
18,000	15.5	13.4	12.0	12.0	11.0	9.5	8.9	8.5
20,000	16.3	14.1	12.6	12.6	11.5	10.0	9.4	8.9
				Critical Distance (feet)				

Note. Reprinted with permission of Arthur Boothroyd.

However, the longer the delay, the more difficult it is to understand speech for listeners with normal hearing as well as those with hearing loss. These challenges have been well documented over the years. We can get a better idea of what is happening if we look at the role frequency plays with reverberation. Looking at the absorption coefficients in Table 3–1, we can see that many of the commonly used building materials affect sounds of different frequencies. Materials like acoustic tile, carpet, and thick curtains absorb high-frequency sounds better than low-frequency sounds. Figure 3–14 illustrates the degree of sound absorption across

frequencies. Treating a room with carpet, acoustic tile, and curtains is common and results in the reduction of reverberation of high-frequency sounds, or the high-frequency components of speech.

Figure 3–14 illustrates some common building materials that absorb more low-frequency sound. Notice that the degree of absorption in Figure 3–14 is much greater than the degree of absorption in Figure 3–15. We can infer from these figures that it is more difficult to absorb low-frequency sound than high-frequency sound. This typically results in more low-frequency sounds reverberating in a listening environment. With

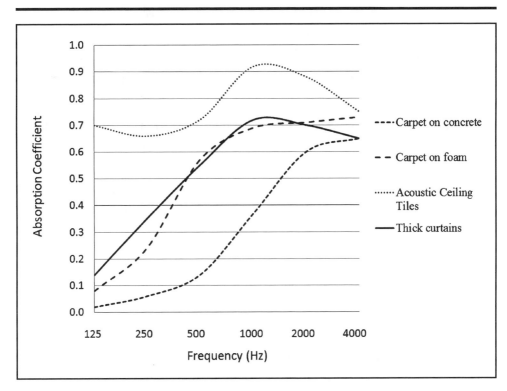

Figure 3–14. Absorption properties of a few common building materials as a function of frequency. Notice that the high-frequency sounds are absorbed more by these materials than the low-frequency sounds.

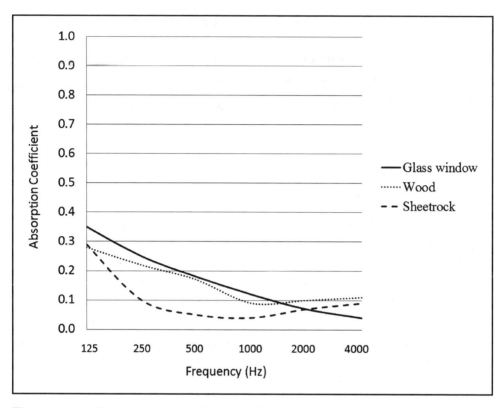

Figure 3–15. The absorption properties of a few common building materials as a function of frequency. Notice that the low-frequency sounds are absorbed more than the high-frequency sounds. Also, notice the degree of absorption. Even though these materials absorb more of the low-frequency sounds, they do not absorb much of them.

more low-frequency sounds reverberating in the listening environment than high-frequency sounds, the difficulty trying to understand speech increases; we know that low-frequency sounds contribute very little to our ability to understand speech and the low-frequency sounds mask the high-frequency speech sounds. The latter is known as the upward spread of masking. These difficulties are exacerbated by high-frequency hearing loss.

In Figure 3–16, we see a speaker and a listener with only some indication of the reverberation, illustrated by the circles and/or curved lines. In Figure 3–16A, the listener is within the critical distance and will have a better chance of understanding the speaker than the listener in Figure 3–16B.

These examples are simplified to illustrate the role of reflected versus direct sound energy in listening. A listener can be beyond the critical distance and remain within the same room as the speaker. We can expand this idea to other challenging listening environments, such as those of listening while in a stairwell and a hallway. Trying to understand speech in a

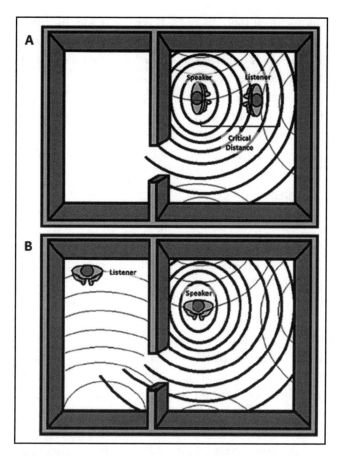

Figure 3–16. A. Looking down into two rooms in which the listener is within the critical distance to the speaker. The majority of the sound energy reaching the listener is coming directly from the speaker. A listener within the critical distance will have a better chance of understanding the speaker. **B.** A view in which the listener is beyond the critical distance to the speaker. The majority of the signal reaching the listener is reflected energy. The listener can be in the same room and still be beyond the critical distance.

stairwell is very difficult, because stairwells are commonly constructed of steel and concrete with large, flat surfaces. The stairwell will likely have longer reverberation times, which results in excessive low-frequency energy. In addition to the poor acoustics for understanding speech, the listener has limited ability to use visual cues or else risk falling down a flight of stairs. Listening in hallways is not much better than listening in a stairwell. The options available to the listener to improve communication include, but may not be limited to, guessing what was said, walking very close to the speaker to stay inside the critical distance, postponing the conversation until all parties are in a more suitable location, or using some form of an assistive listening device.

Noise

In acoustics, noise is thought of as a complex aperiodic signal that spreads energy across many frequencies. However, for anyone trying to listen to someone speaking, noise is any unwanted signal. It is unwanted because it competes with the speech signal for the listener's attention. So, we may find it easier to think of the speech signal that a listener is trying to hear, and any other sounds as competition for the listener's attention.

Noise, or the unwanted/competing signal, can be that complex aperiodic signal that spreads energy across many frequencies mentioned previously. This type of noise is generated from devices and machinery that we interact with in our everyday lives. Whether it is a generator running, car revving, or fan blowing, noise is part of almost every listening environment. Unfortunately, much of this noise is either low frequency in nature or is facilitated by the acoustic characteristics of the environment, such as reverberation. Consequently, the low-frequency components of the noise persist longer and with greater energy than the high-frequency components. Because of this preponderance of low-frequency noise,

there is a greater likelihood of the upward spread of masking. This means that the low frequencies can and will mask (i.e., drown-out) the high frequencies. This is particularly troublesome for those with hearing loss in the high frequencies. Figure 3–17 illustrates the intensity of noise as a function of frequency for a modern passenger vehicle. Of the three conditions, (1) inside the vehicle with the engine off, (2) inside the vehicle with the engine running at idle, and (3) outside the vehicle with the engine running at idle, each has a considerable degree of low-frequency noise. We would likely see similar frequency representation in almost any common listening environment.

Beranek, Blazier, and Figwer (1971) suggested ranges of preferred noise levels to include: (1) no more than 30 dBA SPL (e.g., the intensity of a faint whisper or a quiet library) for large auditoriums, large theaters, and churches; (2) no more than 42 dBA SPL for small auditoriums, small theaters, small churches, music rehearsal rooms, large meeting and conference rooms; and (3) no more than 47 dBA SPL for places to rest or sleep, such as bedrooms, hospitals, small apartments, hotels, motels, or for places where conversation between only a few people is expected, like private offices, small conference rooms, and living rooms. Figure 3–18 illustrates the difference between a quiet listening environment and a noisy environment.

Unfortunately for those with hearing loss, the use of hearing aids does not resolve the problems associated with noise. In Chapter 4, we will see how the processing of background noise in hearing aids has improved in recent years. Yet,

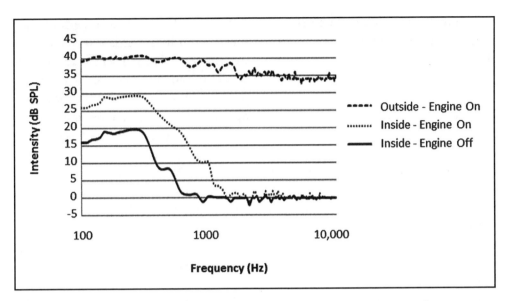

Figure 3–17. The intensity of noise as a function of frequency in a modern passenger vehicle, measured in three conditions: (1) inside the vehicle with the engine off, (2) inside the vehicle with the engine running at idle, and (3) outside the vehicle with the engine running at idle.

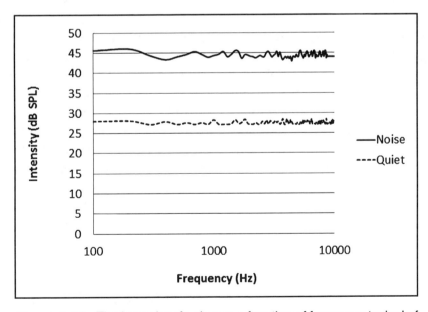

Figure 3–18. The intensity of noise as a function of frequency typical of a relatively quiet room with and without a noise source. Within this room, the noise added came from a small, 8-inch fan.

background noise is one of the chief complaints of hearing aid wearers (Kochkin et al., 2010).

Signal-to-Noise Ratio

Anyone who has tried to hold a conversation in a noisy place knows that the presence of noise can make it difficult to hear. The level of the speech signal compared to the level of the background noise, including the reflected speech signal, is referred to as the signal-to-noise ratio (SNR). When the level of the signal is greater than that of the noise, the SNR is indicated by a positive sign before the amount of the difference. Conversely, a negative sign denotes that the level of the noise is greater than that of the signal. With a large positive SNR, it is quite easy to understand the signal. However, if the level of the noise increases or the level of the signal decreases, we have greater difficulty understanding speech (Nabelek & Pickett, 1974). For satisfactory communication, the level of the signal needs to be at least 6 dB (+6 dB SNR) above the level of the noise (Moore, 1989). These difficulties understanding speech associated with challenging SNRs are exacerbated by those with hearing loss (Nabelek & Mason, 1981) and for children and the elderly (Helfer & Wilber, 1990; Nabelek & Robinson, 1982).

Acceptance of Noise

It is important to understand how well a listener can understand speech under different SNRs (i.e., speech performance measures in noise). It is also valuable to determine at what SNR a listener will surrender the attempt to understand speech in noise, or speech preference measures. Speech preference can be assessed by using the acceptable noise level (ANL) test.

The ANL measures the maximum level of background noise a listener is willing to accept before abandoning the effort to follow the speech. The listener is asked to adjust the maximum level of background noise they judge to be acceptable while listening to speech (Nabelek, Tucker, & Letowski, 1991). The average ANL falls between +10 and +12 dB for adults and between +8 and +10 dB for children (Bryan, Franklin, Ware, & Horne, 2013; Franklin, Thelin, Nabelek, & Burchfield, 2006; Freyaldenhoven & Smiley, 2006). This can be interpreted as adult listeners prefer to listen to speech in noise with a SNR of about +10 to +12 dB, while children prefer a SNR of about +8 to +10 dB. There is a slight difference in the SNR (≈6 dB) that listeners need for satisfactory communication and agreement between the SNR listeners prefer (≈12 dB). Thus, there may be listening situations in which a listener can understand speech, even if it is at a challenging SNR but will give up the attempt at listening because the SNR is below their ANL.

Visual Cues and Barriers

To this point, this chapter has discussed primarily acoustics. It is also worth our time and effort to think about some visual aspects related to hearing. To some degree, most of us rely on visual information when listening to another person. The assistance of seeing a speaker's face is of greater benefit to listeners with hearing loss, as the listener has a better opportunity to gain more information from two inputs, acoustic and visual. Challenges associated with the use of visual cues can involve the relative position of the speaker and the listener. If the speaker has a light source illuminating from behind, the speaker's face will be in the shadow of the speaker's head (e.g., outdoors, a speaker has the sun shining from behind, becoming a hindrance instead of a contribution when the sun shines on the speaker's face). This results in greater difficulty seeing and using visual cues by the listener. As with listening, the use of visual cues is dependent on distance. Visual cues are most accessible when the listener is near the speaker with both the speaker and the listener facing each other. Other challenges to using visual cues may result from a person speaking with food in his or her mouth or with excessive facial hair. On occasion, a speaker may attempt to speak to a person who is located in a different room. Issues related to sound absorption and reverberation can be exacerbated by the lack of visual information.

Summary

In this chapter, we discussed how sound, the transfer of energy across an elastic medium, interacts (i.e., how sound is reflected, transmitted, diffracted, and absorbed) with objects in our surroundings. Part of this interaction includes the original sound signal interacting with itself after being reflected off an object's surface. These interactions result in noisy and reverberant listening environments. This chapter also provided some information about the acoustic characteristics of the speech signal needed to understand speech and differentiate one speech sound from another. The challenge for listeners is to use these small acoustic variations between different speech sounds while in a noisy and reverberant listening environment. It is not easy, but it is exceptionally challenging for those with hearing loss, children, and the elderly. This chapter addressed the difference between a SNR considered to be needed for satisfactory communication and a maximum acceptable SNR (i.e., acceptable noise level). Finally, this chapter addressed the importance of using visual cues when listening. The concepts presented in this chapter should provide a brief introduction both to acoustics and to some of the challenges associated with listening in noisy and reverberant environments. It may be useful to return to this chapter after completing other chapters in this book to review these concepts and challenges.

References

Beranek, L., Blazier, W., & Figwer, J. (1971). Preferred noise criterion (PNC) curves and their application to rooms. *Journal of the Acoustical Society of America*, 50(5A), 1223–1228.

Bryan, M., Franklin, C., Ware, K., & Horne, R. (2013). Acceptable noise levels in preschool children with normal hearing. *Journal of the American Academy of Audiology, 24*(9), 823–831.

Franklin, C., Thelin, J., Nabelek, A., & Burchfield, S. (2006). The effect of speech presentation level on acceptance of background noise in listeners with normal hearing. *Journal of the American Academy of Audiology, 17,* 144–146.

Freyaldenhoven, M., & Smiley, D. (2006). Acceptance of background noise in children with normal hearing. *Journal of Educational Audiology, 13,* 27–31.

Helfer, K., & Wilber, L. (1990). Hearing loss, aging, and speech perception in reverberation and noise. *Journal of Speech, Language, and Hearing Research, 33,* 149–155. doi:10.1044/jshr.3301.149

Kent, R., & Read, C. (1992). *The acoustics analysis of speech.* San Diego, CA: Singular.

Kochkin, S., Beck, D., Christensen, L., Compton-Conley, C., Fligor, B., Kricos, P., . . . Turner, R. (2010). MarkeTrak VIII: Customer satisfaction with hearing aids is slowly increasing. *Hearing Journal, 63*(1), 11–19.

Lass, J. (1996). *The principles of experimental phonetics.* St. Louis, MO: Mosby.

Moore, B. (1989). *An introduction to the psychology of hearing.* San Diego, CA: Academic Press.

Nabelek, A., & Mason, D. (1981). Effect of noise and reverberation on binaural and monaural word identification by subjects with various audiograms. *Journal of Speech, Language, and Hearing Research, 24*(3), 375–383.

Nabelek, A., & Pickett, J. (1974). Monaural and binaural speech perception through hearing aids under noise and reverberation with normal and hearing-impaired listeners. *Journal of Speech, Language, and Hearing Research, 17,* 724–739. doi:10.1044/jshr.1704.724

Nabelek, A., & Robinson, P. (1982). Monaural and binaural speech perception in reverberation for listeners of various ages. *Journal of the Acoustical Society of America, 71*(5), 1242–1248.

Nabelek, A., Tucker, F., & Letowski, T. (1991). Toleration of background noises: Relationship with patterns of hearing aid use by elderly persons. *Journal of Speech and Hearing Research, 34,* 679–685.

4

Hearing Aids and Implantable Devices

The Starting Point for Hearing Assistive and Access Technologies

Hearing Aids and Implantable Devices

Hearing aids, like those in Figure 4–1, or implantable devices often come to mind when the subject of a conversation concerns hearing loss or hearing assistive and access technology. Furthermore, many think of hearing aids and implantable devices as the final step in hearing assistive and access technology. This limited vision of available assistance is understandable as these devices play a signifi-

cant role in assisting those with hearing loss. However, they are only a starting point and the foundation for the rest of this book.

This chapter discusses some benefits of hearing aids and implantable devices. For readability, this chapter focuses more on hearing aid technology; however, much of this technology is applicable to both hearing aids and implantable devices. The chapter provides information related to the improvement in technology, along with the advantages and some limitations of using these devices.

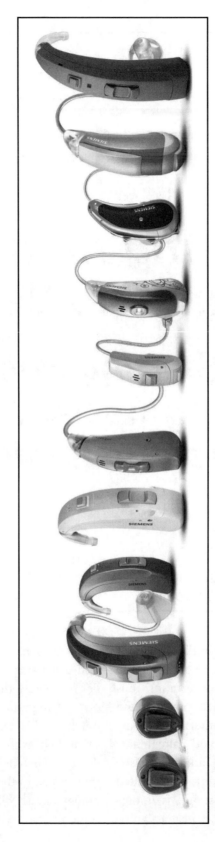

Figure 4–1. Lineup of the sleek design of modern hearing aids. Image courtesy of Siemens.

When you consider that the number of individuals in the United States with hearing loss is over 34 million, and growing, it is quite easy to understand the need to assist these individuals. Presently, the rate of hearing aid acceptance is only approximately 25% (Kochkin, 2009). Thus, there are many individuals who do not use, but could benefit from hearing aids. Hearing aids in one form or another have been in existence for over a century. While many advances and improvements have been made, hearing aids still have a stigma attached to them. It seems that everyone knows someone who has had some sort of problem with their hearing aids (e.g., the hearing aids squeal and feedback too often or at inopportune times, the hearing aids make me look old or disabled, the hearing aids are uncomfortable in and/or on my ears, loud sounds are too loud, background noise is too bothersome). Many of these complaints are warranted. Unfortunately, many people do not realize the strides made to resolve these issues. Hearing aids have transformed from simple mechanical devices to sophisticated digital devices. Contemporary reports indicate that hearing aid wearers find improvement in a number of listening situations. Figure 4–2 provides a number of listening situations in which hearing aid users indicate improvement with the use of hearing aids.

Amplification devices have the primary task of converting acoustic energy (i.e., sound) into a signal that is perceptible to the user. In the case of hearing aids, a hearing aid converts sound into an electric/digital signal, amplifies the signal, and converts the signal back to sound, which is now more intense than the original sound. The conversion of one form of energy to another is referred to as *transduction*. Thus, any mechanism that converts or transduces energy from one form to another is called a *transducer*. Figure 4–3 illustrates the basic path of conversion/transduction, amplification, and a return conversion/transduction. Implantable hearing aids and bone-anchored devices function in a similar manner, but differ slightly as to how the sound is delivered (e.g., driving the ossicles or vibrating the skull). Cochlear implants (CIs) and auditory brainstem implants (ABIs) convert sound into an electrical signal and deliver that signal to the central auditory nervous system.

Hearing aids have advanced from large boxes, too heavy to move from location to location with ease, to tiny devices worn in or on the ear, or even implanted, which are only minimally perceived by the wearer and those interacting with the wearer. With the development of digital processing, the digital signal can be manipulated in a multitude of ways. Advanced signal processing (ASP) has led to the initiation of open canal devices and feedback cancellation, frequency lowering, digital noise reduction, sound scene analysis, datalogging, and artificial intelligence. ASP has improved the functionality of directional microphones and wireless communications as well as size issues.

Although the majority of individuals with hearing loss receive benefit from hearing aids, there are a number of individuals with hearing loss who are better suited using an implantable device.

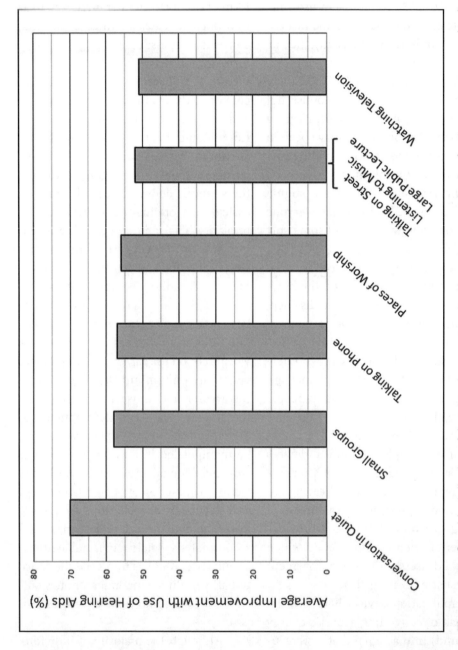

Figure 4–2. Graphical display of the situations and their respective percentages for the greatest perceived hearing handicap improvement with the use of hearing aids. Data from Kochkin, S. (2011). MarkeTrak VIII: Patients report improved quality of life with hearing aid usage. *The Hearing Journal, 64*(6), 25–32.

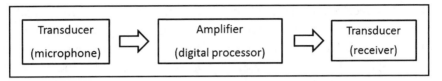

Figure 4–3. The basic processing of a hearing aid, from transduction, through amplification, back to transduction.

Cochlear implants, auditory brainstem implants, and bone-anchored implants provide these individuals with assistance where acoustic hearing aids cannot. As the name *implant* implies, implantable devices require surgery for implantation. Those using bone-anchored implants typically have either a chronic conductive hearing loss (i.e., a problem with the middle and/or outer ear), a mixed hearing loss (i.e., middle and/or outer ear problems along with inner ear problems), or a combination of a severe sensorineural hearing loss (i.e., problem with the inner ear) in one ear with relatively normal hearing in the other ear. This combination is often referred to as single-sided deafness (SSD). Figure 4–4 illustrates a bone-anchored implant device.

Candidacy for cochlear implants depends on a few factors. Depending on the age of the individual, sensorineural hearing loss ranging from moderate to profound is the first factor. Next, the

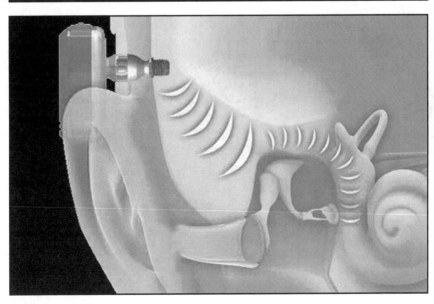

Figure 4–4. A bone-anchored device. Courtesy of Cochlear Americas, © 2014 Cochlear Americas.

candidate must receive only limited benefit from hearing aids as confirmed from a short trial period. The use of auditory brainstem implants is rare as their primary use is to help individuals diagnosed with Neurofibromatosis Type II (NF2), a genetic disorder associated with noncancerous tumors affecting the auditory nerve. Figure 4–5 illustrates a cochlear implant.

Hearing Aid Styles

Contemporary hearing aids come in a variety of sizes and shapes. Early electronic hearing aids were the size of a small suitcase; the idea of carrying these large devices from location to location is daunting. Today, the smallest hearing aids are the size of the tip of your small finger, or smaller. Typically, the names for the different styles of hearing aids are indicative of their size and shape. Hearing aids that sit behind the ear and extend via a tube or wire to the ear canal are referred to as behind-the-ear (BTE) hearing aids. Traditional BTE hearing aids are large and somewhat noticeable to others, due to a thick tube and large earpiece, known as an earmold. However, some BTE hearing aids are considerably smaller than traditional BTE hearing aids with a thin tube or thin insulated wire running to the ear canal. These BTE hearing aids are referred to as open-fit or open-canal hearing aids and consist of two categories, slim tube and receiver-in-the-canal (RIC) hearing aids. The slim-tube, open-canal hearing aids are similar to traditional BTE

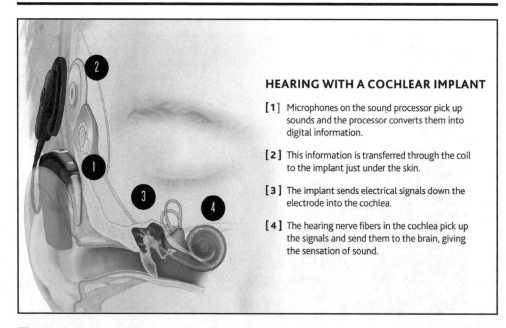

HEARING WITH A COCHLEAR IMPLANT

[1] Microphones on the sound processor pick up sounds and the processor converts them into digital information.

[2] This information is transferred through the coil to the implant just under the skin.

[3] The implant sends electrical signals down the electrode into the cochlea.

[4] The hearing nerve fibers in the cochlea pick up the signals and send them to the brain, giving the sensation of sound.

Figure 4–5. A cochlear implant. Courtesy of Cochlear Americas, © 2014 Cochlear Americas.

hearing aids, as they contain all of the electronic components within the portion that sits behind the ear. Receiver-in-the-canal hearing aids, also referred to as receiver-in-the-ear (RITE) hearing aids, differ from slim-tube hearing aids, as the receiver (i.e., loudspeaker) portion resides in the canal, not behind the ear. Hearing aids that sit in the ear are referred to as in-the-ear (ITE) hearing aids. The names of the styles of ITE hearing aids are typically descriptive of their size, shape, and specific location. The styles include, but are not limited to, full shell, half shell, in-the-canal (ITC), completely-in-the-canal (CIC), invisible-in-the-canal (IIC), and a few other variations of these names. Figure 4–6 illustrates many different styles of contemporary hearing aids.

Compression and Expansion

While it is not in the purview of this chapter to provide an in-depth description of the workings and processing scheme rationales of amplitude compression in both hearing aids and implantable devices, an introductory look at compression is provided. The most common description of amplitude compression typically states that the goal of compression is to take the range of sounds in the listening environment and compress them into the reduced audible of the hearing aid user. In other words, amplitude compression prevents amplified sounds from being amplified beyond the hearing aid wearer's tolerance level and/or attempts to preserve a sense of normal loudness. Compression

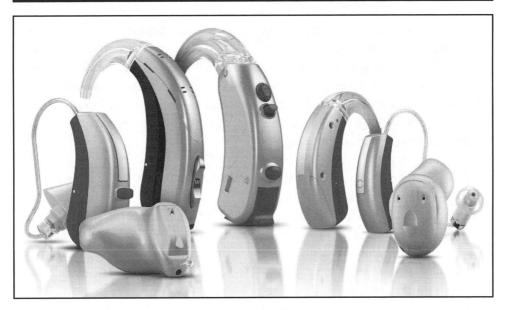

Figure 4–6. Contemporary series of styles of hearing aids with two in-the-ear (ITE) hearing aids in the front row and five behind-the-ear (BTE) hearing aids in the back row. The range of styles varies among hearing aid manufacturers. Image courtesy of Widex.

can be used as a safety feature, such that no amplified sound will cause discomfort or further damage to the auditory system. Thus, very intense sounds get compressed to protect the hearing aid wearer from the loud sound. Compression can also be used to maintain the normal loudness of sound. Thus, amplitude compression attempts to make almost every sound, soft or loud, remain soft or loud for the hearing aid wearer. This process, often referred to as loudness normalization, attempts to keep soft sounds in the listening environment soft, but audible for the hearing aid user, while keeping loud sounds in the listening environment loud, but tolerable for the hearing aid wearer.

After these two basic goals of amplitude compression, there is considerable debate over the optimal method of compressing sound to improve listener comfort and the ability to understand speech. Implementation of compression processing schemes often involves complex combinations of varying attack and release times with multichannel processing. Attack and release times of a compressor refer to the time required for the compressor to take action, or compress the signal, and the time needed to release the signal from being compressed. These times typically vary with the characteristics of the sound needing to be compressed. For very brief environmental sounds, such as a dropped dish onto a hard surface, a fast attack time is preferred. For instances when the speech signal needs to be compressed for comfort and normal loudness, a slower attack is often used in an effort to preserve timing cues used to understand speech. Multi-

channel compression refers to the ability to apply these different processes for different frequency bands. For example, very loud, low-frequency sounds, which hold very little information for understanding speech, may be compressed differently than loud, high-frequency sounds, which contribute greatly to the hearing wearer's ability to understand speech.

Expansion acts in a similar manner as amplitude compression, except that expansion focuses on very soft sounds, such as soft levels of noise or the noise produced by the hearing aid itself. For the purposes of this chapter, expansion may be thought of as a method of reducing soft, unimportant nonspeech sounds from becoming a distraction to the hearing aid wearer. Neither amplitude compression nor expansion provides improved speech understanding for the hearing aid wearer. Some expansion settings may even cause greater difficulty understanding speech than having no expansion processing (Plyler, Hill, & Trine, 2005). In general, these forms of signal processing can be thought of as providing a more comfortable and safer listening experience.

Noise Reduction

With or without hearing aids or implantable devices, understanding speech in a noisy environment can be challenging. When we listen to speech, there will always be accompaniment by some type and degree of background noise. This speech and noise mixture can be thought of as a signal corrupted by noise. Modern hearing aids are capable of removing some of the noise from the signal during signal processing. Before a hearing aid can remove or reduce noise from the mixture of speech and noise, the device must be able to distinguish speech from noise. In order to do this, the characteristics of the speech signal and those of the background noise must be contrasted with one another. These differences allow for a greater likelihood of correct identification of which part of a signal is speech and which part is nonspeech noise. At this point, efforts can be made to remove the nonspeech noise from the mixed signal, leaving only the speech portion of the signal to be amplified.

Because the characteristics of speech often differ from those of noise, the sound scene (i.e., listening environment) can be analyzed based on these differences. Sound scene analyzers typically divide environmental sounds into three or four categories including, but not limited to noise, speech-in-noise, speech (i.e., speech-in-quiet), and quiet. These analyzers typically categorize sounds using techniques such as modulation depth, modulation analysis, and spectral analysis. Modulation depth refers to the fluctuations in signal intensity. Characteristically, the intensity level of speech changes quickly from one speech sound to another, whereas nonspeech noise typically maintains a relatively consistent level (e.g., the noise floor). An illustration of modulation depth is provided in Figure 4–7. Calculating modulation depth provides some of the information needed to accurately differentiate speech from nonspeech.

Modulation analysis assesses the rate of modulations of a sound. That is, it provides additional information to assist in differentiating speech from nonspeech as noise typically has a much higher modulation rate than speech. Synchrony analysis, focusing only on high-frequency components of a sound, looks for harmonic patterns, which are indicative of speech.

Once the sound scene analysis is performed and speech can be differentiated from nonspeech, different methods of signal processing can occur. One form of signal processing is digital noise reduction (DNR). The complaint about listening to speech when noise is present is common among hearing aid wearers. Reducing the noise from the signal should allow for better speech understanding in noisy listening environments. Despite the intent of DNR to enhance speech perception, it has shown very little, if any, capacity for this; hearing aid wearers typically prefer DNR, as it results in more comfortable listening, which ultimately leads to increased hearing aid use. It can be argued that DNR results in indirect improvement in speech communication (Bentler & Mueller, 2011).

Another use of sound scene analysis is datalogging and artificial intelligence. Datalogging is a record of the amount of time a hearing aid has been worn for total use and in different listening environments (i.e., quiet, noise, speech-in-noise, speech-in-quiet). Datalogging can provide some insight into the hearing aid wearer's patterns of use and help the hearing aid learn the wearer's preferences in each listening situation. This learning and automatic adjustment is a form of artificial intelligence and has the potential to provide more ease and convenience to the hearing aid wearer.

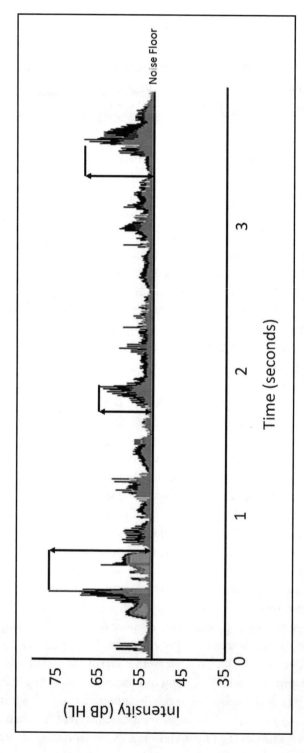

Figure 4–7. Speech with changing modulation depth for the phrase, "Her pluck and grit have writ her name in crimson flame." The noise floor is represented by a straight black line with constant intensity level of 52 dB and little to no variability. The speech phrase, shown as areas of gray and black, reveals the constantly varying modulation depth of peak and valleys between 52 and 70 dB HL.

Directional Microphones

Another hearing aid and implantable device feature intended to improve the signal-to-noise ratio (SNR) for the hearing aid wearer is the directional microphone. Presently, hearing aids employ two types of microphone arrangements to provide either directional or omnidirectional sensitivity. Omnidirectional microphone arrays are designed to have uniform sensitivity to sounds in all directions, while directional microphone arrays provide variable sensitivity based on direction. Typically, directional microphones are more sensitive in front of the wearer, assuming that the wearer is looking at the speaker. While there are multi-

ple variations of directional microphones, this chapter focuses on the general concepts, advantages, and limitations related to directional microphones. Figure 4–8 illustrates the sensitivity of a directional microphone. To some degree, the use of contemporary directional microphones improves the SNR for the wearer, improving comfort and speech understanding (Lurquin & Rafhay, 1996; Valente, Fabry, & Potts, 1995; Wouters, Litière, & van Wieringen, 1999). Even though there has been debate regarding the appropriateness of employing directional processing for children, directional microphones contribute to better understanding in noise for children (Gravel, Fausel, Liskow, & Chobot, 1999; Kuk, Jackson, Keenan,

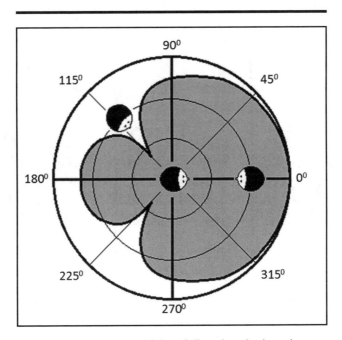

Figure 4–8. The sensitivity of directional microphones. The microphones are more sensitive to the person in the shaded area in front of the listener than the person behind the listener.

& Lau, 2008). The effectiveness of directional microphones is limited in listening situations in which the speaker is at a distance farther than the immediate vicinity of the hearing aid wearer, such as beyond the critical distance for reverberation. Any advantage due to directional microphones for listening in such situations is diminished. In addition, hearing aid patients often report a preference for the loudness perceived when the hearing aids are in an omnidirectional microphone mode over directional mode (Bentler & Mueller, 2011; Wu & Bentler, 2010a, 2010b). Directional microphones have also shown some promise in localizing

a sound source. O'Brien, Yeend, Hartley, Keidser, and Nyffeler (2010) found that directional microphone use improved the ability of the hearing aid wearer to distinguish between high-frequency (i.e., 2000 to 5000 Hz) sounds coming from in front of versus behind the listener.

Modern hearing aids now have directional sensitivity, which is automatic (i.e., the hearing aid adapts the directional mode based on the listening situation and/or environment). This adaptive directionality is intended to facilitate listening in situations where the wearer is not able to face the person speaking, for example, while driving a car (Figure 4–9).

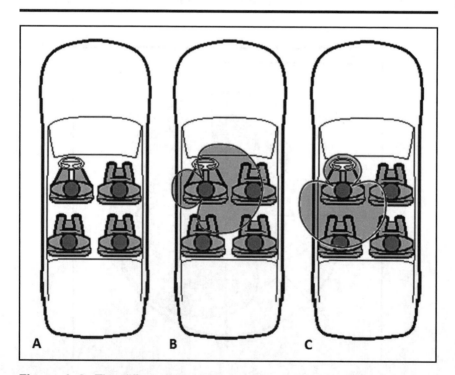

Figure 4–9. The difference in adaptive directional processing in a challenging listening situation, such as driving a car. **A.** The sensitivity of a "fixed" directional microphone. **B** and **C.** The sensitivity of directional microphones designed to adapt to whomever is speaking.

This feature makes the directional mode depend on an accurate sound scene analyzer. If the hearing aid does not accurately classify the listening environment, the effect of the directional microphone could be minimized. Even if the listening environment is classified accurately, there are variables such as input signal level and type of sound that trigger the adaptive directionality that must be considered (Bentler & Mueller, 2011). With the exception of a few situations, there is little, if any, additional benefit of adaptive directionality over fixed directionality in real-world listening environments (Woods, Merks, Zhang, Fitz, & Edwards, 2010). There is the potential for significantly better directional microphone benefit with improvement in technology. The use of microphones from two hearing aids fit binaurally and communicating wirelessly with each other has the potential to improve directional effects. This technology has been named "super directional microphones" (Beck, 2013).

Even though there have been improvements in this technology, it is important to recognize some of the limitations of directional microphones. While directional microphones improve speech intelligibility in the presence of noise, they provide little, if any, improvement in reverberant listening situations (Hoffman, Trine, Buckley, & Van Tasell, 1994). Also, although directional microphones deliver a good amount of additional benefit to the hearing aid wearers, the benefit from this technology is not as important as using visual cues (Bentler & Mueller, 2011; Wu & Bentler, 2010a, 2010b).

Remote Microphones and Wireless Communication

Many individuals with hearing aids and implantable devices use wireless technology to interface with remote microphones, mobile phones, televisions, or multimedia (e.g., Bluetooth, infrared systems, induction loop, and FM systems). Issues related to telephone use with hearing aids have improved with wireless communication. Historically, the communication between the hearing aid and telephone existed via an induction loop system. This system employs a magnetic field, generated by a traditional landline telephone, to transmit the signal to a telecoil inside the hearing aid. Recently, advances in wireless technology have allowed for more sophisticated strategies of communicating between telephone and hearing aid. Hearing aid telephone features vary among manufacturers. Some modern hearing aids receive the telephone signal and transmit that signal to only the hearing aid being used with the telephone while turning down the volume of the second hearing aid. This volume adjustment allows the hearing aid on the ear using the telephone to have an advantage over the hearing aid on the nontelephone ear, while allowing the nontelephone hearing aid to still provide some amplification of sounds in the proximity of the hearing aid wearer. Such wireless communication also allows for an alternate strategy, in which the hearing aid wearer is able to hear the telephone signal in both ears for an improved listening situation. In this case, the hearing aids on both sides of the head receive the signal. While improving the ability to understand what is being spoken over the phone, this strategy reduces the hearing aid wearer's ability to hear or detect sounds in their immediate surroundings.

Wireless communication between telephones and hearing aids has advanced beyond the mere signal transmitter–signal receiver relationship. This wireless communication has expanded to include mobile smart devices communicating with hearing aids. Presently, many hearing aids can be adjusted or controlled via smart devices to maximize listener preference. These adjustments include adjusting the volume setting, changing from directional to omnidirectional microphone modes, and changing programs designed for different listening environments. Chapters 6 through 9 have more information regarding wireless communications and wireless communications with hearing aids and implantable devices.

Like directional microphones, remote microphones allow hearing aid wearers and those with implantable devices to hear and understand more speech in noisy environments including when several talkers are present. A remote microphone refers to a microphone that is positioned within a separate device. This device can be placed near the sound source, such as in front of a speaker's mouth. Remote microphones have an advantage over directional microphones; remote microphones facilitate better hearing and understanding of speech over a greater distance than present directional microphones, usually 30 feet or more. Remote microphones are much less susceptible to interference due to reverberation and other background noise between the speaker and the hearing aid wearer, because a remote microphone is placed close to the speaker's mouth, essentially moving the listener's ear to that location, too. Figure 4–10 illustrates one of the remote microphones presently available to hearing aid wearers.

Frequency Lowering

The primary goal of frequency lowering is to make inaudible speech sounds audible.

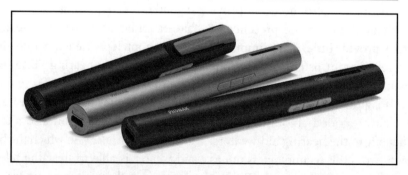

Figure 4–10. Phonak's discreet-looking Roger Pen acts as a remote microphone. Use of remote microphones facilitates listening in noisy and reverberant environments. Image courtesy of Phonak.

Frequency lowering is an umbrella term used to describe the processing of a signal in which the high-frequency parts of the speech signal (i.e., high-frequency bands) are represented at lower frequencies (i.e., low-frequency bands). The intent of frequency-lowering schemes is to make high-frequency sounds audible to those with high-frequency hearing loss by shifting those high-frequency sounds to the regions in which the degree of the hearing loss may not be as severe (e.g., lower frequencies). There are a few basic methods of frequency lowering: transposition, compression, and translation (Mueller, Alexander, & Scollie, 2013; Scollie, 2013). The first frequency-lowering technique, frequency transposition, transfers high-frequency sounds down in frequency by an octave or two. Frequency transposition is a linear function; that is, no frequency bands are compressed in the process. The signal processing combines the transposed sound with the original, nontransposed lower-frequency sounds. So, a high-frequency speech sound, like "s," would be transposed into a lower-frequency region (e.g., where the "ch" sound resides). In this scenario, the "s" and the "ch" sounds would overlap each other due to the frequency transposition.

The second technique of frequency lowering, known as frequency compression, is named aptly as it compresses the frequency bands above a designated cutoff frequency into a narrower output range. In a frequency compression process, the high-frequency "th" sound would be compressed along with adjacent lower-frequency sounds, like "g" and "k," to fit both the high- and low-frequency sounds into the frequency range of better hearing. The degree by which compression takes place is defined by the compression ratio.

The next method, frequency translation, only initiates the frequency-lowering process when a high-frequency signal is identified. If a high-frequency sound is detected, frequency translation is initiated and, like frequency transposition, the high-frequency sound is mixed with the low-frequency sound. In addition to transposing the high-frequency sound, frequency translation leaves the high-frequency sound at its original frequency. So, it is represented twice, once at a lower frequency and at its original high frequency. Scollie (2013) refers to frequency translation as adaptive and acting at the "speed of phonemes." In this case, the "f" sound in the word "off" would trigger the frequency translation. The "f" sound would be represented at a lower frequency where "g" resides and also at its original, higher frequency. Conversely, the word "on," which does not have a high-frequency component, would not initiate the frequency translation. The benefits of frequency lowering are probably best observed by those with hearing loss in the high frequencies so severe that the high-frequency portion of the speech signal cannot be amplified enough to make it audible, or the signal is audible but the auditory system is so damaged that it distorts the sound. These individuals, and potentially others, benefit from improved detection and recognition ability of high-frequency speech sounds, like "s" and "sh" (Glista et al., 2009). Figure 4–11 illustrates the configuration of a

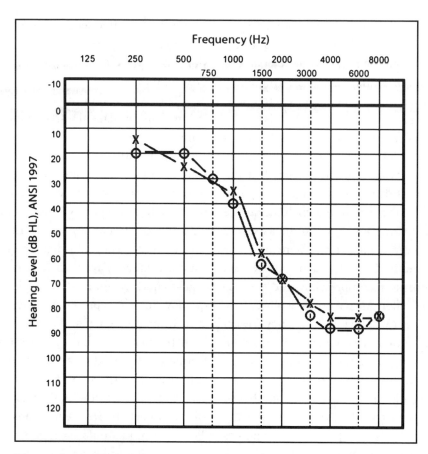

Figure 4–11. The configuration of hearing loss likely to be best suited for frequency lowering.

hearing loss likely suited to benefit from frequency lowering.

Personal Sound Amplification Products

Personal sound amplification products (PSAPs), like hearing aids, are electronic devices designed to amplify sounds in the listening environment. However, according to the Food and Drug Admin-istration (FDA, 2009), only hearing aids are designed with the intent to aid those individuals with hearing loss. Hearing aids are considered medical devices and thus are held to FDA regulations related to safety and effectiveness. Only licensed professionals (i.e., audiologists or hear-ing aid dispensers) can dispense hearing aids. In contrast, PSAPs are designed for individuals with normal hearing while performing specific listening tasks (e.g., watching television without disturbing someone sleeping nearby, listening in lecturers or meetings). This differentiation by the FDA has not deterred those with hearing loss to purchase PSAPs in place of purchasing hearing aids. In fact, a large portion of PSAP purchasers identify themselves as having hearing loss (Kochkin, 2010). While some have argued that PSAPs may serve as a first step toward the purchase of hearing aids by these individuals, Kochkin (2010) reports that less than 18% of PSAP owners with self-professed hearing loss plan to purchase hearing aids. It has been concluded that it is likely these individuals would choose to live without hearing aids if PSAPs were not currently available.

Presently, many PSAPs have the ability to implement wireless communications with smart devices in a manner similar to hearing aids. Many PSAPs can be adjusted via smart devices to maximize listener preference. Because of the association between PSAPs and modern smart devices, many potential hearing aid wearers view the use of PSAPs as more acceptable than the perceived stigma of wearing hearing aids. Figure 4–12 shows a PSAP being worn in the ear.

Summary

This chapter addressed hearing aid styles, processing schemes related to amplitude compression and expansion, the use of directional microphones, remote microphones, wireless, and frequency-lowering technology. Hearing aid styles range in

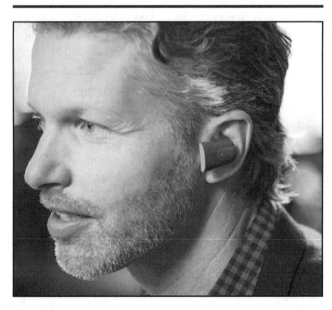

Figure 4–12. Example of a personal sound amplification product (PSAP). Image courtesy of Soundhawk.

size from very small, like the IIC and CIC, to larger BTE hearing aids. Regardless of size, amplitude compression and expansion provide more comfortable and safer listening. In addition, noise reduction processing can, to some degree, determine speech from nonspeech sounds to provide more ease of listening for hearing aid and implantable device users. Directional microphones can improve SNR, often resulting in greater ability to understand speech in noise. Remote microphones improve SNR better than directional microphones, as remote microphones are less susceptible to noise and reverberation. The use of wireless technology is making an impact on hearing aid success. Although wireless technology in hearing aids and implantable devices is in its early stages, this technology has great potential for improving hearing aid and implantable device benefit. Frequency lowering technology attempts to provide the hearing aid wearer access to sounds by shifting the sounds in frequency regions where the hearing loss is the greatest to regions of better residual hearing. Finally, this chapter introduced PSAPs as devices designed for improved listening, other than to aid those with hearing loss. Although hearing aids and implant devices provide assistance to those with hearing loss, each type of technology has some limitations. Together with other hearing assistive and access technologies that form the basis for this book, access to additional auditory, visual, and tactile cues can further promote independence, enhance quality of life, and improve social communication.

References

Beck, D. (2013). *Super directional hearing aids, noise reduction, and APD: Interview with Harvey Dillon, PhD.* Retrieved from http://www.audiology.org/news/Pages/20130214.aspx

Bentler, R. A., & Mueller, H. G. (2011). 20Q: Hearing aid features—The continuing search for patient benefit. *AudiologyOnline.* Retrieved from http://www.audiologyonline.com/

Center for Devices and Radiological Health, Food and Drug Administration. (2009). *Regulatory requirements for hearing aid devices and personal sound amplification products.* U.S. Department of Health and Human Services. Retrieved from http://www.fda.gov/downloads/MedicalDevices/DeviceRegulationandGuidance/GuidanceDocuments/ucm127091.pdf

Glista, D., Scollie, S., Bagatto, M., Seewald, R., Parsa, V., & Johnson, A. (2009). Evaluation of nonlinear frequency compression: Clinical outcomes. *International Journal of Audiology, 48*(1), 632–644.

Gravel, J., Fausel, N., Liskow, C., & Chobot, J. (1999). Children's speech recognition in noise using omnidirectional and dual-microphone hearing aid technology. *Ear and Hearing, 20*(1), 1–11.

Hoffman, M., Trine, T., Buckley, K., & Van Tasell, D. (1994). Robust adaptive microphone array processing for hearing aids: Realistic speech enhancement. *Journal of the Acoustical Society of America, 96,* 759–770.

Kochkin, S. (2009). MarkeTrak VIII: 25 year trends in the hearing health market. *Hearing Review, 16*(11), 12–31.

Kochkin, S. (2010). MarkeTrak VIII: Utilization of PSAPs and direct-mail hearing aids by people with hearing impairment. *Hearing Review, 17*(6), 12–16.

Kochkin, S. (2011). MarkeTrak VIII: Patients report improved quality of life with hearing aid usage. *The Hearing Journal, 64*(6), 25–32.

Kuk, F., Jackson, A., Keenan, D., & Lau, C. (2008). Personal amplification for school-age children with auditory processing disorders. *Journal of the American Academy of Audiology, 19*(6), 465–480.

Lurquin, P., & Rafhay, S. (1996). Intelligibility in noise using multimicrophone hearing aids. *Acta Otorhinolaryngology Belgium, 50*(2), 103–109.

Mueller, H. G., Alexander, J. M., & Scollie, S. (2013). 20Q: Frequency lowering—The whole shebang. *AudiologyOnline*, Article 11913. Retrieved from http://www.audiologyonline.com/

O'Brien, A., Yeend, I., Hartley, L., Keidser, G., & Nyffeler, M. (2010). Evaluation of frequency compression and high-frequency directionality. *The Hearing Journal, 63*(8), 32, 34–37.

Plyler, P. N., Hill, A. B., & Trine, T. D. (2005). The effects of expansion on the objective and subjective performance of hearing instrument users. *Journal of the American Academy of Audiology, 16*(2), 101–113.

Scollie, S. (2013). 20Q: The ins and outs of frequency lowering amplification. *AudiologyOnline*, Article 11863. Retrieved from http://www.audiologyonline.com/

U.S. Food and Drug Administration. (2013). *Consumer health information.* Retrieved from http://www.fda.gov/downloads/ForConsumers/ConsumerUpdates/UCM373847.pdf

Valente, M., Fabry, D., & Potts, L. (1995). Recognition of speech in noise with hearing aids using dual microphones. *Journal of the American Academy of Audiology, 6*(6), 440–449.

Woods, W., Merks, I., Zhang, T., Fitz, K., & Edwards, B. (2010). Assessing the benefit of adaptive null-steering using real-world signals. *International Journal of Audiology, 49*, 434–443.

Wouters, J., Litière, L., & van Wieringen, A. (1999). Speech intelligibility in noisy environments with one- and two-microphone hearing aids. *Audiology, 38*(2), 91–98.

Wu, Y. -S., & Bentler, R. A. (2010a). Impact of visual cues on directional benefit and preference: Part 1—Laboratory tests. *Ear and Hearing, 31*(1), 22–34.

Wu, Y. -S., & Bentler, R. A. (2010b). Impact of visual cues on directional benefit and preference: Part 2—Field tests. *Ear and Hearing, 31*(1), 35–46.

5

Needs Assessment

Introduction

There are several facets to assessing the needs of an individual with hearing loss, including the audiologic evaluation of hearing sensitivity and auditory system integrity, speech understanding in quiet and noise, the effects of hearing loss on the psychosocial state of the individual, daily communication, communication at home, communication at the workplace (if applicable), and social activities, for a start. There are also some aspects of the individual that impact the treatment and management of hearing loss (e.g., readiness of the client to make changes in their life, their locus of control, and their quality of life). Research of these topics in audiology has begun in the last 10 to 15 years, and there are some interesting and informative results, shared later in the chapter.

In this chapter, we first have a brief overview of the World Health Organization's framework of *International Classification of Functioning, Disability and Health* (ICF; 2002). The elements of this model are (1) health condition, body structure, and functions; (2) activity limitations; (3) participation restrictions; (4) environmental factors; and (5) personal factors. We use these areas to think about what constitutes a thorough needs assessment. Note that in audiology, the terms *client* and *patient* are often used interchangeably. Many audiologists do not work in medical settings and therefore *client* was chosen for use.

The World Health Organization's *International Classification of Functioning, Disability and Health*

We begin this section by mentioning a WHO classification schema that many are likely familiar with, the *Classification of Diseases* or the ICD series (e.g., ICD-9). The medical coding used by health care professionals for diagnosis and billing in the United States was developed by the WHO. Audiologic examples of ICD-9 codes are sensorineural hearing loss-389.18; dizziness-388.70 and acoustic trauma-388.11. The ICF is a similar idea that provides a classification system of health and health-related domains (WHO, 2014b). The WHO is certainly one of the primary, if not the primary, recognized world leaders in the health care arena for influencing the [world's] health research agenda, developing and disseminating norms and standards, making clear the health care evidence-base and policy options that evidence supports, delivering technical assistance in health care to countries, among others (WHO, 2014a). In recognition of the global leadership and transnational nature of the WHO, the "World Health Assembly," a legislative body for the WHO with representatives from each member state, formally votes on and adopts documents such as ICF and ICD-9. The current ICF was adopted as the "international standard to describe and measure health and disability" (WHO, 2014b).

What is meant by a classification system of health and health-related domains? At heart the ICF is a framework for including disability as a part of the human existence continuum. To create this new model of disability, the ICF authors melded two older views: the *social model* of disability and the *medical model* of disability. Historically these two somewhat opposing models have been used to think about, treat, and work with individuals with disabilities and their environments. In the *social model,* society and the environment are understood to cause an individual's difficulties and the problems are not caused by any particular characteristic(s) of the person. For example, think about a person with a mobility issue in an older building. She uses a wheelchair and needs to get to an office on the third floor of this building that was built in 1913, and that has an elevator too small for the wheelchair to fit into. In the *social model,* this situation would be characterized as a societal problem because the physical environment does not accommodate all persons in the society. As we saw in Chapter 2, the Americans with Disabilities Act (ADA, 1990, 2008) went a long way to addressing these types of physical environment issues, but before 1990, the various and differing needs of individuals with disabilities were not necessarily taken into consideration for building design and physical accessibility. In the *medical model,* the thinking is that the individual has a "problem" that needs to be treated and managed, or treated and cured, individually by a medical professional. Those subscribing to the *medical model* do not necessarily recognize that a person's environment is an important component that should be addressed, although there seems to be a growing appreciation of that fact in the larger medical community. It seems clear that both models, as far as each one goes, has merit; the difficulty is that the component(s) not recognized as important within each model also have merit. Thus, the WHO led a process to address this lack of coherence into a single, viable model of disability by combining the *social* and *medical* models into a *biopsychosocial model*. An introductory (WHO, 2002) explanation of the biopsychosocial model is provided at http://www.who.int/classifications/icf/icfbeginnersguide.pdf?ua=1. An important point of this model is the idea that it is a biopsychosocial one, recognizing the complex interactions among the body (bio), the mind/disposition (psycho), and a person's physical and peopled environments (social). It follows, then, that audiologists would do well to perform a complete needs assessment—that is, evaluate their clients in each of the sections of the ICF model. The various pieces of this model (Figure 5–1) for a client with hearing loss, that client's

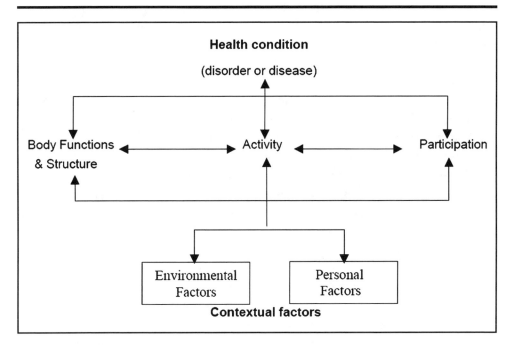

Figure 5–1. ICF model of health and health-related domains. Reproduced, with the permission of the publisher, from *Towards a Common Language for Functioning, Disability and Health: ICF The International Classification of Functioning, Disability and Health.* World Health Organization (2002). Retrieved from http://www.who.int/about/en/

life situation, and the client's abilities to function in his or her environment are described as follows.

The *health condition* is the hearing loss. *Body structures* refers to the affected anatomical portions that factor into the condition (e.g., outer hair cell loss in the cochlea or fused bones in the middle ear). *Body functions* refer to the abilities of the auditory system, given the damaged or malfunctioning body structures. *Activities* are just that—what tasks or actions the person can perform. *Participation* has a broader meaning and includes events and situations that the individual can engage in. Stated in this way, *activities* and *participation* are defined in a positive way—that is, what the individual can do. However, in practice, we speak about *activity limitations*, or problems the individual has to complete tasks, and *participation restrictions*, difficulties the individual experiences while in particular situations. Contextual factors has two components, *environmental factors* (the physical world of the person, the society and that society's ethos, mores, and laws) and *personal factors* (e.g., age, sex, coping style, education, profession, life experience, character, and how the person experiences the disability).

There are several additional points to be made about this model. First, note that each component is interdependent with every other component. What does that mean? Practically speaking, that means a change in any one component could cause changes in all the others, in either a positive or negative direction, or both. Another characteristic of the ICF model is that it classifies three human functioning levels: (1) body or body part, (2) whole person, and (3) whole person in a social context (WHO, 2002). In school, audiologists are taught that we are treating the person, not the hearing loss. The interdependent nature of the components of the ICF model coupled with the recognition of factors at these three levels should reinforce that message, and also make us think that the situation may be even more complex than we originally thought. The key is that we perform an adequate needs assessment that addresses each of the components in the ICF model. We turn to the needs assessment now.

Needs Assessment

Before we think about particular tests, instruments, and questions we might use in our assessment, we want to acknowledge an important idea connected with treating clients: *patient- and family-centered care* (PFCC). Although PFCC is not a new concept, it has received increased attention by the health care industry in recent years. The overarching concept of PFCC is that the client and her/his family should be included as team members in all aspects of the client's health care, from being given accurate, timely, and unbiased information, to developing and carrying out the treatment plan. Individuals and families may participate to whatever degree they feel comfortable with, which we, as professionals, should honor. In audiology, we have long recognized how important it is to include family members and other communication partners in the treatment process; this renewed emphasis on PFCC in the larger health care context is simply a good reminder for us to continue to do that. In fact, such involvement of the client and family, as well as the WHO-ICF, has been recognized by the American Academy of Audiology (AAA) in its *Guidelines for the Audiologic Management of Adult Hearing Impairment* (Valente et al., 2006). Valente et al. state:

■ The combined efforts of the audiologist, client, significant others, and/or caregivers are essential.

■ In keeping the WHO-ICF, assessment is viewed as a multifaceted process, including assessment of auditory function to diagnose the extent of the impairment; assessment of activity limitations and participation restrictions through self-report of communication need and performance; assessment of environmental and personal contextual factors; and consideration of how all the levels of assessment impact QOL . . .

■ . . . The use of technology other than hearing aids, referred to as "hearing assistive technology" (HAT), should be part of the process. (p. 4)

Likewise, the American Speech-Language-Hearing Association (ASHA) has developed and published preferred practice patterns which speak to all aspects of this needs assessment, including the audiologic evaluation, basic amplification, audiologic rehabilitation (AR), hearing assistive technology systems (HATs), and outcome evaluation and follow-up measures (ASHA, 2006). We encourage reading these practice pattern documents, which each include "Expected Outcomes," "Clinical Indications," and "Clinical Process."

Assessing Health Condition, Body Structures, and Body Functions

We now discuss the evaluation of a person with hearing loss within the WHO-ICF model. The basic audiologic evaluation is the instrument audiologists use to perform these assessments, beginning with the case history. Portions of the case history, in addition to providing information about the health condition, body structures, and body functions, might also provide information about each of the other components of the WHO-ICF, depending on which questions the audiologist/clinic includes in the basic history. In terms of the health condition and body, the case history will likely have questions about the individual's hearing status, tinnitus status, medical conditions, and medications that may influence the person's hearing. The first two of these, hearing and tinnitus status, are important to provide the individual's self-assessment of the impact of those on their person. The latter two have increased in importance given the growing body of evidence that sensorineural hearing loss (SNHL) occurrence is associated with, for example, cardiovascular risk factors (Helzner et al., 2011) and early-onset type 2 diabetes mellitus (Lerman-Garber et al., 2012), and that sudden SNHL is correlated with increased risk of acute myocardial infarction (Lin et al., 2013) and diabetes mellitus (Lin et al., 2012). Furthermore, audiologic case history data that, historically, have been thought to tell us about the person's environment (exclusively) may actually also inform us about aspects of the person's hearing health/medical condition(s). For example, noise-induced SNHL, long known as the only preventable etiology of hearing loss, may be exacerbated in individuals who work in noise and are exposed to repetitive vibrations such as from construction tools (Palmer et al., 2002) and certain chemicals (Hodgkinson & Prasher, 2006; Vyskocil et al., 2012). Additionally, the available information related to genetically based conditions resulting in hearing loss, or which have hearing loss as a possible component, is growing exponentially. In the areas of genetics and medications, audiologists simply must be aware of and determine, if presented with an unfamiliar genetic condition or medication, the effects of those on the audiologic system. We note in the appropriate section(s) additional information from the case history that will help inform us about the WHO-ICF.

All elements of the basic audiologic evaluation provide us information about a person's audiologic (health) condition and anatomic structures and functions, as noted in Tables 5–1 and 5–2. And, clearly, specialized audiologic tests provide additional information on more targeted anatomic/functional areas.

Audiologists are quite skillful at determining the state of a person's audiologic system with our extensive diagnostic capabilities. The key is to leverage that information and gather the appropriate pieces of other relevant information to provide sufficient and helpful nonmedical treatment. What "other" information is relevant? Minimally, we need to understand the impact of a person's hearing status on his or her daily life, social interactions, work setting, recreational endeavors, and other communication situations that are important to him or her as an individual. What information do audiologists already typically obtain? How does that information fit within the WHO-ICF framework for environmental and personal factors, and how do those factors interact with and influence the individual's activity limitations and participation restrictions?

Assessing Environmental Factors

When we think of *environmental factors* we need to be careful to distinguish the "environment" (i.e., conditions that are external to the person, and the "situation," the person's perception of the environment). While the environment can be objectively described, the situation is, by its nature, the subjective reality for the individual and is best thought of in the WHO-ICF model under Personal Fac-

Table 5–1. Audiologic Structure or Function Evaluated by Standard Audiometric Procedure

Procedure	Structure/Function
Otoscopy	Pinna, ear canal, eardrum
Tympanometry	Middle ear
Otoacoustic emissions	Outer hair cells
Pure tone testing	Cochlea, behavioral response to sound
Acoustic reflexes	Acoustic reflex arc (middle ear, cochlea, portions of the VIIth and VIIIth cranial nerves)
Speech reception threshold; word recognition testing	Cochlea, central auditory nervous system VIIIth cranial nerve

Table 5–2. Audiologic Structure or Function Evaluated by Special Audiometric Procedure

Procedure	Structure/Function
Auditory brainstem response	Inner hair cells and/or IHC-VIIIth nerve synapses, VIIIth nerve
Middle latency responses	Mid-brain, thalamus, cortex
Late latency responses	Cortex
Speech in noise tests	Cochlea, central auditory nervous system, cortex

tors. The person's perceptions will govern how she or he interprets and interacts with the environment and is discussed in the next section.

Audiologists are aware of the importance of understanding our clients' various listening environments, so we ask about the physical environments and the background noise where our clients converse and listen. See Chapter 3 in this volume for a detailed explanation of the effects of the physical environment on listening. Audiologists recognize that the background noise is a combination of at least the sound levels, frequency content of the background sounds, or sound spectra, and reverberation qualities of the physical spaces (see Chapter 3). Also important are the social environments. Some of the information audiologists need to know is who the client's interaction partners are, how much interaction the client has with each of them, and which people in what situations are particularly difficult. An additional question to ask in reference to this last situation is how are those situations and/or people difficult? For example, does a communication partner have facial hair or speak with a hand in front of the face, or does he or she speak to our client with the back turned or from a separate room? Audiologists provide information, often handouts, on techniques to improve communication with difficult communication partners and/or in noisy environments.

A client's home is a very important listening space. Just as important are the social activities such as church, synagogue, or mosque attendance; theater; and get-togethers with friends, either in the friends' homes or in public spaces. What is some basic information audiologists need to help their clients make informed decisions about personal amplification and hearing assistive technology? Here is a "starter" list of questions, and you are encouraged to add to this list:

- Which situations are difficult for the client to communicate in? Why?
- Does the client listen to the radio or watch television?
- Does the client use a computer, use programs such as Skype or FaceTime?
- Does the client have a landline telephone, mobile phone, both, or neither? How well can the client use each of those devices? What causes difficulties?
- If there is no telephone in the home, a referral to your state's "telephone assistance program" is a must. Although the names vary, this type of program exists in each state and lends landline telephones to qualifying individuals on a permanent basis.
- What type of mobile phone does the client own? Is it Bluetooth enabled? (Note that the Telecommunications Equipment Distribution Program Association [TEDPA; http://www.tedpa.org] is a good resource to find out about your state's program. In 2014 Delaware, Michigan, New York, and Washington, DC, did not have state-wide programs, according to TEDPA.)
- If the client attends religious services, does that institution have hearing assistive technology available? Is the space looped? (Note that looping for telecoil use has become quite popular again in some states. It may be wise to find out what venues in your city have this capability and place a telecoil in personal amplification devices.)
- Does the client attend live theater, movie theaters, the symphony, or go to museums? What hearing assistive technology is available at each of these places?

With working-age clients, one environmental situation that needs focused attention during the needs assessment is the workplace, not only the physical environment, which includes what the office looks like and what materials it is made from, but also the social environment of the workplace and the client's job functions. It is likely that the client will need assistive devices in the workplace, and our job is to understand his or her job functions, as well as the physical and social environments in order to make the most appropriate recommendations with respect to amplification and/or hearing assistive technology. Audiologists rarely, if ever, travel to a client's home or workplace to obtain information about the physical space. One way to acquire good information about the physical environment is to have the client bring photographs (e.g., taken with his or her mobile phone) to an audiology appointment of work and home spaces important to their communication. This information should aid the audiologist in determining, for example, telephone to computer connections, if needed, and what type of assistive and access technology would work best in the conference room. Many of the same questions as above will be useful in this context. The audiologist may want to obtain details about which situations and communication partners (if any) cause the most difficulty for the client and begin by addressing those.

A very important idea to keep in mind is this: clients may have little to no knowledge about hearing assistive/ access technology and what devices are available to help them in their day-to-day lives. It is the responsibility of audiologists to teach clients about this important aspect of hearing health care.

Assessing Personal Factors

What does "personal factors" mean? The WHO-ICF describes personal factors as gender, age, coping styles, social background, education, profession, past and current experience, overall behavior pattern, and character. That is quite a list, but audiologists often routinely collect some pieces of information that help inform us about the ICF personal factors, including gender, age, profession, past and current experience (but that is often limited to experience with hearing aids), and perhaps education. If we undertake hearing aid and/or audiologic rehabilitation consultation, we may ask about social background (i.e., what social activities do the client and significant others engage in). The pieces we generally do not ask about are coping style, behavior pattern, and character. The authors suspect that most audiologists do not see these characteristics (coping style, behavior pattern, character) as information we should ask the clients about. The fact that there are only a few studies in the literature with regard to these traits might support that. However, in the last 10 to 15 years two research groups, notably Cox, Alexander, and Gray (1999, 2005, 2007) and Laplante-Levesque, Hickson, and Worrall (2010, 2011, 2012, 2013) have undertaken systematic study of several personal factors including perceived degree of disability, locus of control, self-efficacy, coping style, personality, and stages of change.

The research in this area of personal factors and their influence on an individual with hearing loss are based partially on the Transtheoretical Model of Change (TTM) (Prochaska & DiClemente, 1983). An explanation of this model is beyond the scope of this book; however, several constructs of TTM (locus of control, self-efficacy, stages of change) have been validated for a number of health-related activities. These activities include physical exercise (Jones et al., 2013), smoking cessation (DiClemente et al., 1991), and changes in diet (Greene et al., 1999), among many others.

We encourage learning about this important theoretical framework for behavior change because the work of Cox et al. and Laplante-Levesque et al. and others, demonstrates that the TTM constructs are relevant for people with hearing loss. These researchers report that compared to a person with hearing loss who does not seek amplification, a person seeking amplification (1) has a greater perceived level of hearing disability (Laplante-Levesque et al., 2011, 2012); (2) is at a greater contemplation stage of change, that is, more ready to make a change in his or her life (Laplante-Levesque et al., 2011, 2012); (3) has a more internal locus of control, meaning he or she feels personally powerful in dealing with life's challenges (Laplante-Levesque et al., 2011, 2012); (4) has lower communication self-efficacy denoting lower confidence that he or she can perform a specific behavior (Cox et al., 2005); and (5) may be more routine oriented and less

likely to think of creative ways to manage hearing loss (Cox et al., 2005).

Those clients who report having a successful intervention outcome tend to have higher self-reported hearing disability as well as higher disability perceived by others (Laplante-Levesque et al., 2011, 2012), have a lower precontemplation stage of change and greater action stage of change (they admit there is a problem and are willing to do something about it; Laplante-Levesque et al., 2011, 2012), and have a lower chance locus of control—they do not think life events are random, they think that they and others can influence the outcome of events (Cox et al., 2005).

These are important questions about clients that audiologists historically have not asked. More research must be done to better understand all the personal factors that are important in hearing health care decisions. Even without additional research, however, the Ida Institute has online tools available now to help audiologists and their clients engage in meaningful conversations. These conversations can lead to both parties understanding what a client is thinking in relation to seeking hearing health care and what the audiologist can do to assist the client in decision making. The Ida Institute, based in Copenhagen, Denmark, is a nonprofit organization that focuses on promoting living well with hearing loss as well as tools designed to help professionals and clients move toward that goal. The Ida Institute states on its homepage: "We share and co-create knowledge and tools with hearing care professionals to help them open communication with patients and better address their needs" (http://ida institute.com/).

Tools From the Ida Institute

There are many tools available on the Ida Institute website, but we present only three. It is important to note that these tools are grounded in many of the same constructs as the TTM and are designed to help the audiologist elicit exactly the information discussed above. The first tool, *The Line* (Figure 5–2), can help an audiologist discover whether improving hearing is important to a client and if a reluctant client is ready to take action (stages of change). Further, does the client have access to the resources to perform the recommended treatment? These resources are likely monetary but may also be related to coping style, personality, and social network. Last, is the client confident about using amplification (self-efficacy)? Using this tool, the audi-

ologist can come up with many relevant questions and have the client respond by marking a location on the line.

The Box (Figure 5–3) is intended to facilitate a discussion of a client's ambivalence about getting help for the hearing loss. The client may be unaware of his or her own thoughts, whether positive or negative, in this area; use of the Box may reveal those. Client motivation level can also be explored with the Box and the client can be encouraged to become more active in and move forward with hearing loss treatment.

The Circle (Figure 5–4) is a graphic representation of the (seven) stages of change mentioned previously. Note that "precontemplation" is located outside the "work" area to indicate the person has not self-identified as having any problem and, therefore, does not need to change any behavior(s). Knowing where our client is on the Circle will let us know when the client is ready to make changes and

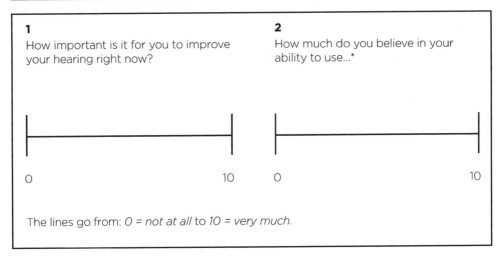

Figure 5–2. The Line. Courtesy of the Ida Institute.

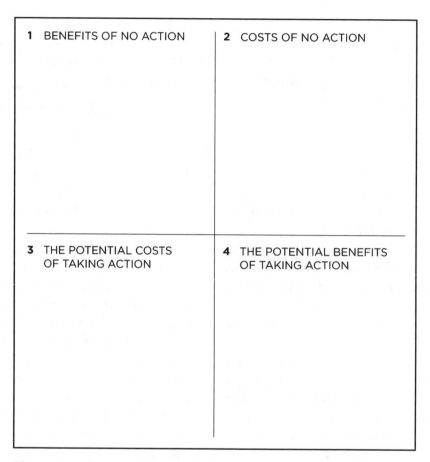

1 BENEFITS OF NO ACTION	2 COSTS OF NO ACTION
3 THE POTENTIAL COSTS OF TAKING ACTION	4 THE POTENTIAL BENEFITS OF TAKING ACTION

Figure 5–3. The Box. Courtesy of the Ida Institute.

also when the client is ready to hear various types of information. That knowledge allows the audiologist to adjust recommendations as needed.

Assessing Activity Limitations and Participation Restrictions

Recall that in the ICF model activity limitations and participation restrictions are separate pieces, and in the model represent different aspects of how the individual interacts with his or her environment. The ICF model defines *activity* as "the execution of a task or action by an individual," and *participation* as "involvement in a life situation" (WHO, 2002, p. 10). For an individual with a disability that limits physical mobility, this activity versus participation distinction works well. The distinction may be less clear, however, when we think about hearing loss because the impact of communication is so wide-reaching. That is not to say that audiologists cannot or should not use this

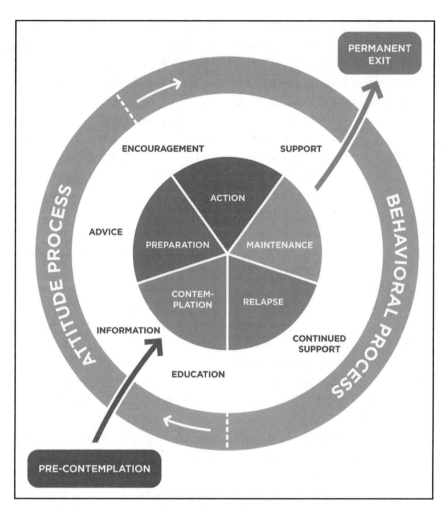

Figure 5–4. The Circle. Courtesy of the Ida Institute.

model, only that we need to be flexible in our application of the model. Let's think about some examples of activity limitations and participation restrictions that may be relevant for someone with hearing loss.

A hearing loss may make using the telephone difficult or not possible, which is an activity in the WHO-ICF framework. Thinking about that particular activity, what situations (i.e., what participation) could be jeopardized for the individual? Some of these might be communicating with family members who are geographically separated, particularly when a computer with some type of video (e.g., Skype or FaceTime) is not available, or placing an emergency call. A quite common complaint is, of course, understanding speech in the presence of background noise (activity). Think about how many situations may be compromised if understanding in background noise is an issue for a client. The answer is almost every situation, given that we spend most of our time in places with sounds that are not the sound of interest, making them "background noise."

Given this situation with hearing loss, it may be less important for audiologists to delineate whether a client's difficulty should be categorized as an activity or as participation than it is for the audiologist to understand the particular situations that are difficult for each client. Therefore, we recommend that audiologists spend enough time with a client to develop a good understanding of the particular settings that cause the client trouble, as well as the particular components of those settings that cause difficulty. One does not need a specialized tool to collect this information; simple conversation and note-taking will suffice. However, there are instruments such as the Client Oriented Scale of Improvement (COSI) (Dillon, James, & Ginis, 1997), the Compton Assistive Technology Questionnaire (Compton, 2000), and the Communication Questionnaire (Morris, 2007) that are designed to help the client think about these issues. To use the COSI, the audiologist and client identify up to five situations that cause the client trouble. The client first prioritizes the situations and estimates the percentage of understanding they experience with no intervention (e.g., hearing aids, audiologic rehabilitation program). The intervention is applied and at a follow-up visit the client and audiologist talk through each situation, discussing whether any improvement in understanding occurred

in those situations once the intervention occurred. The Compton Assistive Technology Questionnaire and Morris' Communication Questionnaire allow for a more holistic approach to evaluate one's life and needs related to hearing loss and not only specific situation identification, as does the COSI. All of these instruments are useful to the audiologist as a way to begin to understand the challenges of their clients.

There are several other self-assessment tools available to audiologists to gather information either pre- and post-intervention or only postintervention. Several of these are the *Speech, Spatial and Qualities of Hearing Scale* (Gatehouse & Noble, 2004), *Satisfaction with Amplification in Daily Life* (Cox & Alexander, 1999), the *Abbreviated Profile of Hearing Aid Benefit* (Cox & Alexander, 1995), and the *Device Oriented Subjective Outcome Scale* (DOSO) (Cox, Alexander, & Xu, 2014). The DOSO is an interesting addition to the literature for at least two reasons. First, Cox and her colleagues designed this tool to measure hearing aid outcomes in a way that is hearing aid wearer personality independent. This development is important because personality is one of the personal factors included in the ICF model and has been shown to influence hearing health care outcomes, as discussed earlier. Second, the areas assessed by the DOSO (speech cues, listening effort, pleasantness, quietness, convenience, and use), may help identify areas in which hearing aids alone are insufficient and additional assistive hearing technologies will help the client.

Assessing Compensatory Strategies

Everyone with hearing loss develops particular ways to converse, interact with family, get spoken information, and listen to TV and music. Audiologists must discover which compensatory strategies are used and, based on the utility of those strategies, either reinforce those behaviors with the client and family or help the client and family come up with better ones. Table 5–3 lists some of the strategies clients and their communication partners may adopt.

These few strategies are not meant to be comprehensive. Rather, these strategies are offered as a starting point for the audiologist to engage with clients and communication partners in a discussion of how they have adapted to the hearing loss. We suggested earlier that discussing various listening situations would be fruitful to planning treatment and want to reiterate that point here, as the strategies adopted may vary by situation.

Table 5–3. Compensatory Strategies Adopted by People With Hearing Loss and Their Communication Partners

Person With Hearing Loss	Helpful	Not Helpful	Helpful	Not Helpful	Communication Partner
Lip/speech reading	✓		✓		Get attention of person with hearing loss
Ask for repetition/rephrase	✓		✓		Face the person with hearing loss
Ask for clarification	✓		✓		Speak clearly
Turn down/off background sounds	✓		✓		Speak slowly
Positions speaker's face in a light source	✓		✓		Provide the topic
Tell others of communication problems	✓		✓		Rephrase (do not repeat)
Avoid conversation		✓	✓		Use keywords
Dominate conversation		✓	✓		Ask for confirmation of information
Bluff understanding (e.g., nods, smiles)		✓		✓	Shout
Blame others for communication difficulty		✓		✓	Shout from a different room

Outcome Measures

Strictly speaking, performing outcome measures with clients may not be part of the needs assessment process. However, if audiologists do not document whether their treatment strategies with a client result in a noticeable difference in the client's life, we have not served that client to the fullest. A second reason we must obtain outcome measures is that in the new and swiftly changing health care arena, third-party payers want evidence that the professional has made a positive difference in the client's life.

How might we evaluate client outcomes? There are two broad categories of outcome measures: objective and subjective. Objective measures include items such as percent correct on a speech in noise test while subjective measures are those in which the client's perceptions are recorded. Self-report measures of benefit from and satisfaction with amplification include the *Abbreviated Profile of Hearing Aid Benefit* and the *Satisfaction with Amplification in Daily Life*.

A more global concept for an outcome measure that is fairly new for audiology is q*uality of life* (QoL). The World Health Organization's Quality of Life group defines QoL as "a broad multidimensional concept that usually includes subjective evaluations of both positive and negative aspects of life." Said another way, a QoL measure is an individual's perception of how he or she is doing. Several instruments have been designed to assess QoL, and more specifically health-related quality of life (HRQoL), such as the *Short Form-36 Health Survey* (SF-36), the *Activities of Daily Living* (ADL), and the *Health Utilities Index* (HUI). Many generic HRQoL instruments such as the ones mentioned have no or only one to two questions about hearing loss which, necessarily, are broad and do not provide enough information about the impact of hearing loss on the individual.

The American Academy of Audiology (AAA) convened a task force to perform a systematic review of the literature on HRQoL and the use of amplification in adults. The task force's conclusions are that, in fact, generic HRQoL instruments capture little effect of hearing aid use on quality of life but that hearing loss specific questionnaires do, including the *Hearing Handicap Inventory for the Elderly* (Ventry & Weinstein, 1982), *Hearing Handicap Inventory for Adults* (Newman, Weinstein, Jacobson, & Hug, 1990), and the *Quantified Denver Scale of Communication Function* (Tuley, Mulrow, Aguilar, & Velez, 1990). The task force reported the use of hearing aids reduces the negative psychological, social, and emotional effects of sensorineural hearing loss in adults. Other research groups, using instruments about communication ability, hearing threshold data, and generic HRQoL questionnaires, have shown that in older adults, greater levels of hearing loss are associated with lower HRQoL results (Chia et al., 2007; Dalton et al., 2003). Chia et al. (2007) also found slightly higher HRQoL scores for people who wear hearing aids on a consistent basis versus those who do not.

There are also instruments designed specifically for those with hearing loss who receive cochlear implants: the *Nijmegen Cochlear Implant Questionnaire* (Hinderink, Krabbe, & Van Den Broek, 2000), the *Patient Quality of Life Form* (Mo, Lindbaek, & Harris, 2005), and the *Index Relative Questionnaire Form* (Wexler, Miller, Berliner, & Crary, 1982). The *Performance Inventory for Profound Hearing Loss Answer Form* (Owens & Raggio, 1988) is not specific for cochlear implant recipients. Loeffler et al. (2010) reviewed studies of these four hearing loss–specific and two generic QoL instruments (SF-36 and the HUI) in individuals with cochlear implants. In general, across-study results suggest that generic instruments are not sensitive enough to changes in perceived quality of life in individuals with cochlear implants and that condition-specific QoL instruments do capture changes.

The important information about quality of life measures is that there are already hearing loss–specific measures available that demonstrate QoL changes of our clients. Audiologists should consider incorporating at least one of these measures into every client's treatment program in order to document that our treatment results in improved outcomes for our clients. For those individuals who do not report improvement with hearing aids, for example, that information is evidence that other avenues should be explored: hearing assistive technologies, audiologic rehabilitation, and auditory training, to name a few.

There are two new QoL instruments designed for children and adolescents with hearing loss, the *Hearing Environments and Reflection on Quality of Life* (HEAR-QL) questionnaire (Umansky, Jeffe, & Lieu, 2011) and the *Youth Quality of Life-Deaf and Hard of Hearing* (HQOL-DHH) questionnaire (Patrick et al., 2011). With many QoL instruments for children with chronic conditions, caregivers must fill them out. However, each of these instruments is designed to be self-administered, the HEAR-QL for children aged 7 to 12 and the HQoL-DHH for adolescents aged 11 to 18. Umansky et al. report the HEAR-QL distinguishes between children who do and do not have hearing loss, and suggest this is an appropriate choice of outcome measure to evaluate interventions for children with hearing loss. The authors of the HQoL-DHH report this instrument has three domains: self-acceptance/advocacy, perceived stigma, and participation. The QoL results were correlated with the Children's Depression Inventory, which was associated with all three domains in the expected direction. Good reliability and validity to assess hearing-specific QoL in adolescents were measured for the HQoL-DHH. Interestingly, no difference in results is reported for teens with differing degrees of hearing loss. More recent work on the same instrument (Meyer et al., 2013) reveals differences on the HQoL-DHH in all three domains between teens with severe to profound hearing loss who use no technology or cochlear implants versus those with hearing aids. Such a tool could be quite enlightening and useful to audiologists who work with adolescents, as particular areas of need can be measured rather than inferred from conversations or otherwise.

Summary

In this chapter we have introduced the World Health Organization's International Classification of Functioning, Disability and Health as the framework within which a needs assessment of individuals with hearing loss can occur. The areas to assess include health condition, body structures, and body functions, which are all done within the context of the audiologic evaluation. Additional areas for assessment are activity limitations and participation restrictions, and within the domain of communication may see overlap. The final areas to assess are environmental factors and personal factors. Audiologists have long recognized and assessed environmental factors; some aspects of the personal factors may be new for audiologists to think about and assess, for example, locus of control and self-efficacy. To help with assessing personal factors, we introduced tools produced by the Ida Institute, a good resource for audiologists regarding the psychosocial aspects of hearing loss. Finally, in the assessment is determining what compensatory strategies the client and communication partner(s) have adopted, and counsel as appropriate. Outcome measures are important both to ensure the best care for clients and also as evidence of client improvement for third-party payers.

References

ADA Amendments Act of 2008, Pub. L. 110-325, codified as amended at 42 USCA § 12101 note. Retrieved from http://www.eeoc.gov/laws/statutes/adaaa.cfm

American Speech-Language-Hearing Association. (2006). *Preferred practice patterns for the profession of audiology* [Preferred practice patterns]. Retrieved from http://www.asha.org/policy/PP2006-00274.htm#sec1.4.19

Americans with Disabilities Act of 1990, Pub. L. 101-336, 104 Stat. 327 (1990). Retrieved from http://www.gpo.gov/fdsys/pkg/STATUTE-104/pdf/STATUTE-104-Pg327.pdf

Chia, E. M., Wang, J. J., Rochtchina, E., Cumming, R. R., Newall, P., & Mitchell, P. (2007). Hearing impairment and health-related quality of life: The Blue Mountains Hearing Study. *Ear and Hearing, 28,* 187–195.

Compton, C. (2000). Assistive technology for enhancement of receptive communication. In J. Alpiner & P. McCarthy (Eds.), *Rehabilitative audiology* (3rd ed., pp. 501–555). Baltimore, MD: Williams and Wilkins.

Cox, R. M., & Alexander, G. C. (1995). The abbreviated profile of hearing aid benefit (APHAB). *Ear and Hearing, 16*(2), 176–186.

Cox, R. M., & Alexander, G. C. (1999). Measuring satisfaction with amplification in daily life: The SADL scale. *Ear and Hearing, 20*(4), 306–316.

Cox, R. M., Alexander, G. C., & Gray, G. (1999). Personality and the subjective assessment of hearing aids. *Journal of the American Academy of Audiology, 10*(1), 1–13.

Cox, R. M., Alexander, G. C., & Gray, G. (2005). Who wants a hearing aid? Personality profiles of hearing aid seekers. *Ear and Hearing, 26*(1), 12–26.

Cox, R. M., Alexander, G. C., & Gray, G. (2007). Personality, hearing problems, and amplification characteristics: Contributions to self-report hearing aid outcomes. *Ear and Hearing, 28*(2), 141–162.

Cox, R. M., Alexander, G.C., & Xu, J. (2014). Development of the Device Oriented Subjective Outcome (DOSO) Scale. *Journal of the American Academy of Audiology, 25*(8), 727–736.

Dalton, D. S., Cruickshanks, K. J., Klein, B. E. K., Klein, R., Wiley, T. L., & Nondahl, D. M. (2003). The impact of hearing loss on quality of life in older adults. *The Gerontologist, 43*(5), 661–668.

DiClemente, C. C., Prochaska, J. O., Fairhurst, S. K., Velicer, W. F., Velasquez, M. M., & Rossi, J. S. (1991). The process of smoking cessation: An analysis of precontemplation, contemplation, and preparation stages of change. *Journal of Consulting and Clinical Psychology, 59*(2), 295–304.

Dillon, H., James, A., & Ginis, J. (1997). Client Oriented Scale of Improvement (COSI) and its relationship to several other measures of benefit and satisfaction provided by hearing aids. *Journal of the American Academy of Audiology, 8*(1), 27–43.

Gatehouse, S., & Noble, W. (2004). The speech, spatial and qualities of hearing sale (SSQ). *International Journal of Audiology, 43*, 85–99.

Greene, G. W., Rossi, S. R., Rossi, J. S., Velicer, W. F., Fava, J. L., & Prochaska, J. O. (1999). Dietary applications of the stages of change model. *Journal of the American Dietetic Association, 99*(6), 673–678.

Helzner, E. P., Patel, A. S., Pratt, S., Sutton-Tyrrell, K., Cauley, J. A., Talbott, E., . . . Newman, A. B. (2011). Hearing sensitivity in older adults: Associations with cardiovascular risk factors in the Health, Aging, and Body Composition Study. *Journal of the American Geriatric Society, 59*(6), 972–979. doi:10.1111/j.1532-5415.2011.03444.x

Hinderink, J. B., Krabbe, P. F., & Van Den Broek, P. (2000). Development and application of a health-related quality-of-life instrument for adults with cochlear implants: The Nijmegen Cochlear Implant Questionnaire. *Otolaryngology-Head and Neck Surgery, 123*(6), 756–765.

Hodgkinson, L., & Prasher, D. (2006). Effects of industrial solvents on hearing and balance: A review. *Noise Health, 8*, 114–133. doi:10.4103/1463-1741.33952

The Ida Institute. (n.d.). *Motivation tools.* The Ida Institute. Retrieved from http://idainstitute.com/index.php?id=1293#/tool_room/motivation_tools/motivation_tools/?type=1337

Jones, C., Jancey, J., Howat, P., Dhaliwal, S., Burns, S., McManus, A., . . . Anderson, A. S. (2013). Utility of stages of change construct in the planning of physical activity interventions among playgroup mothers. *BMC Research Notes, 6*, 300. doi:10.1186/1756-0500-6-300

Laplante-Lévesque, A., Hickson, L., & Worrall, L. (2010). Factors influencing rehabilitation decisions of adults with acquired hearing impairment. *International Journal of Audiology, 49*(7), 497–507. doi:10.3109/14992021003645902

Laplante-Lévesque, A., Hickson, L., & Worrall, L. (2011). Predictors of rehabilitation intervention decisions in adults with acquired hearing impairment. *Journal of Speech, Language and Hearing Research, 54*(5), 1385–1399. doi:10.1044/1092-4388(2011/10-0116)

Laplante-Lévesque, A., Hickson, L., & Worrall, L. (2012). What makes adults with hearing impairment take up hearing aids or communication programs and achieve successful outcomes? *Ear and Hearing, 33*(1), 79–93. doi:10.1097/AUD.0b013e31822c26dc

Laplante-Lévesque, A., Hickson, L., & Worrall, L. (2013). Stages of change in adults with acquired hearing impairment seeking help for the first time: Application of the transtheoretical model in audiologic rehabilitation. *Ear and Hearing, 34*(4), 447–457. doi:10.1097/AUD.0b013e3182772c49

Lerman-Garber, I., Cuevas-Ramos, D., Valdes, S., Enriquez, L., Lobato, M., Osornio, M., . . . Gomez-Perez, F. J. (2012). Sensorineural hearing loss—A common finding in early-onset type 2 diabetes mellitus. *Endocrinology Practice, 19*(4), 549–557. doi:10.4158/EP11389.OR

Lin, C., Lin, S. W., Lin, Y. S., Weng, S. F., & Lee, T. M. (2013). Sudden sensorineural hearing loss is correlated with an increased risk of acute myocardial infarction: A population-based cohort study. *The Laryngoscope, 123*, 2254–2258. doi:10.1002/lary.23837

Lin, S. W., Lin, Y. S., Weng, S. F., & Chou, C. W. (2012). Risk of developing sudden sensorineural hearing loss in diabetic patients: A population-based cohort study. *Otology & Neurotology, 33*, 1482–1488. doi:10.1097/MAO.0b013e318271397a

Loeffler, C., Aschendorff, A., Burger, T., Kroeger, S., Laszig, R., & Arndt, S. (2010). Quality of life measurements after cochlear implantation. *Open Otorhinolaryngology Journal, 4*, 47–54.

Meyer, A., Sie, K., Skalicky, A., Edwards, T. C., Schick, B., Niparko, J., & Patrick, D. L. (2013). Quality of life in youth with severe to profound sensorineural hearing loss. *Otolaryngology-Head and Neck Surgery, 139*(3), 294–300. doi:10.1001/jamaoto.2013.35

Mo, B., Lindbaek, M., & Harris, S. (2005). Cochlear implants and quality of life: A prospective study. *Ear and Hearing, 26*(2), 186–194.

Morris, R. A. (2007). *On the job with hearing loss: Hidden challenges successful solutions.* Florence, KY: Bluegrass Press.

Newman, C. W., Weinstein, B. E., Jacobson, G. P., & Hug, G. (1990). The hearing handicap inventory for adults: Psychometric adequacy and audiometric correlates. *Ear and Hearing, 11*, 430–433.

Owens, E., & Raggio, M. (1988). Performance Inventory for Profound and Severe Loss (PIPSL). *Journal of Speech and Hearing Disorders, 53*(1), 42–56.

Palmer, K. T., Griffin, M. J., Syddall, H. E., Pannett, B., Cooper, C., & Coggon, D. (2002). Raynaud's phenomenon, vibration induced white finger, and difficulties in hearing. *Occupational and Environmental Medicine, 59*, 640–642.

Patrick, D. L., Edwards, T. C., Skalicky, A. M., Schick, B., Topolski, T. D., Kushalnagar, P., . . . Sie, K. S. (2011). Validation of quality-of-life measure for deaf or hard of hearing youth. *Otolaryngology-Head and Neck Surgery, 145*(1), 137–145.

Prochaska, J. O., & DiClemente, C. C. (1983). Stages and processes of self-change of smoking: Toward an integrative model of change. *Journal of Consulting and Clinical Psychology, 51*(3), 390–395.

Tuley, M. R., Mulrow, C. D., Aguilar, C., & Velez, R. (1990). A critical reevaluation of the Quantified Denver Scale of Communication Function. *Ear and Hearing, 11*, 56–61.

Umansky, A. M., Jeffe, D. B., & Lieu, J. E. C. (2011). The HEAR-QL: Quality of life questionnaire for children with hearing loss. *Journal of the American Academy of Audiology, 22*(10), 644–653. doi:10.3766/jaaa.22.10.3

Valente, M., Abrams, H., Benson, D., Chisolm, T., Citron, D., Hampton, D., . . . Sweetow, R. (2006). Guidelines for the audiologic management of adult hearing impairment. *Audiology Today, 18*(5), 44 pages. Retrieved from http://www.audiology.org/resources/documentlibrary/Documents/haguidelines.pdf

Ventry, I. M., & Weinstein, I. M. (1982). The Hearing Handicap Inventory for the Elderly: A new tool. *Ear and Hearing, 3*, 128–134.

Vyskocil, A., Truchon, G., Leroux, T., Lemay, F., Gendron, M., Gagnon, F., . . . & Viau, C. (2012). A weight of evidence approach for the assessment of the ototoxic potential of industrial chemicals. *Toxicology and Industrial Health, 28*, 796–819. doi:10.1177/0748 233711425067

West, R. L., & Smith, S. L. (2007). Development of a hearing aid self-efficacy questionnaire. *International Journal of Audiology, 46*, 759–771. doi:10.1080/14992020701545898

Wexler, M., Miller, L. W., Berliner, K. I., & Crary, W. G. (1982). Psychological effects of cochlear implant: Patient and "index relative" perceptions. *Annals of Otology, Rhinology and Laryngology, 91*(2 Pt. 3), 59–61.

World Health Organization. (2002). *Towards a common language for functioning, disability and health: ICF The International Classification of Functioning, Disability and Health.* Retrieved from http://www.who.int/about/en/

World Health Organization. (2014a). *About WHO.* Retrieved from http://www.who.int/about/en/

World Health Organization. (2014b). *Classifications.* Retrieved from http://www.who.int/classifications/icf/en/

WHOQOL Group. (1998). The World Health Organization Quality of Life Assessment (WHOQOL). Development and psychometric properties. *Social Science and Medicine, 46*, 1569–1585.

PART II

Technologies for Hearing Enhancement

6

Frequency-Modulated (FM) Systems

Overview

One of the most well-recognized hearing assistive technologies (HATs) is the frequency-modulated (FM) system used to augment hearing. FM systems are grouped separately from two other hearing augmenting HATs, induction loop systems and infrared (IR), which are discussed in Chapters 7 and 8, respectively. Although all three of these systems operate using some wireless mechanism, the FM system appears to be the most versatile of the three because of its flexibility for a number of different listening situations. However, one is not necessarily superior to the others in terms of sound quality provided that the products are of high quality and properly installed or fitted.

Of the three HATs, FM has made the most dramatic changes over the last 40 to 50 years. FM systems have commonly been used in the educational setting for children with hearing loss. The teacher wears a microphone/transmitter, and the student with hearing loss wears a receiver. There are many who recall when FM systems had a body worn receiver device held to the chest using buttoned straps around the waist and shoulders (Figure 6–1). The output of this device was delivered to one or both ears through wires up to older snap-on, button-style receivers with custom earmolds. Teachers wore a lavalier-style microphone/transmitter (not pictured in Figure 6–1), which was also quite large and bulky. In the past, these FM systems were called *auditory trainers* when the student wore a single unit that served both as hearing aid and FM

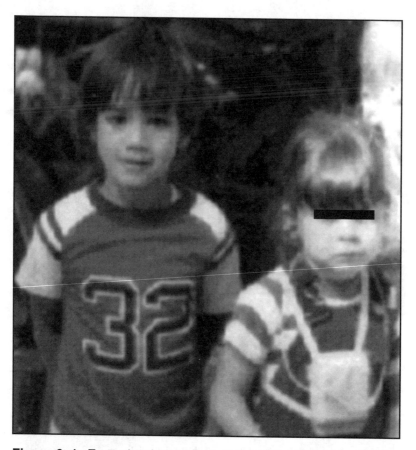

Figure 6–1. Example of an older body-worn frequency-modulated (FM) system often referred to as an auditory trainer (*child on the right*). A teacher nearby [not in photograph] is wearing a lavalier-style microphone transmitter. One of the authors wearing his own hearing aids is the small boy on the left. Photo courtesy (circa 1979) of Samuel R. Atcherson, PhD.

receiver. Anecdotal reports by others who remember wearing these body-worn FM receivers were wearing them as late as the mid-1990s, just 20 years ago.

Today, some of the most advanced FM systems have been integrated (built-in) directly into personal hearing aids; alternatively, there are small FM audio shoes that can be attached directly onto many hearing aids and implantable devices. The microphone/transmitter has also enjoyed some miniaturization and is now generally small enough to clip on a belt, place in a pocket, or wear around the neck, so long as the microphone is within about 6 inches of the teacher's mouth. With a common one-way transmission range of up to about 100 feet (though some much farther), the FM receiver and microphone/transmitter can be separated and used in different locations, such as on different floors or in different cars. There are also soundfield amplification systems that operate using FM transmission. Here, for example, the teacher wears a microphone, and the signal is sent to a receiver amplifier and a loudspeaker to be projected acoustically throughout a room. In this chapter, we describe FM technology, discuss its various applications, and provide practical information to maximize its use.

What Is FM?

Recall from Figure 1–1 that FM is one of several wireless systems using discrete electromagnetic radiation frequency bands for transmission of audio signals. Similar to FM radio stations used for

commercial broadcasting of news and music, two special frequency regions, 72 to 76 MHz and 216 and 217 MHz, were authorized and allocated for use as carrier frequencies for HATs by the Federal Communications Commission (FCC). In contrast to IR and induction systems, which use light and magnetic signals, respectively, FM uses radio frequencies. As the name implies, the transmission of audio frequencies is modulated by a carrier frequency (i.e., within the 72 to 76 or 216 to 217 MHz regions) in a manner that the wavelengths become longer or shorter as the audio signal frequency changes. (Figure 6–2 provides a comparison of frequency modulation versus amplitude modulation.) In addition, as the center frequency of the carrier deviates up and down (e.g., moves from 72.4 to 72.5 MHz), the audio signal intensity (soft or loud) is represented. Thus, the transmission from the FM microphone/transmitter to the FM receiver is indeed

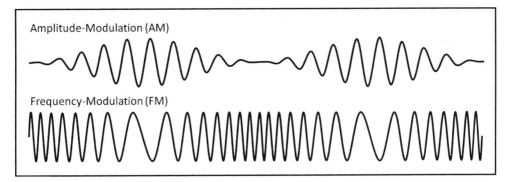

Figure 6–2. Comparison of amplitude modulation (AM) and frequency modulation (FM). While both signals have changing patterns, AM changes in amplitude but not frequency, while FM changes in frequency, but not amplitude. Note that the intensity (loudness) of FM signals is conveyed by moving the carrier frequency up or down.

a radio-frequency signal. The transmitter combines (modulates) the carrier and audio frequencies, while the receiver disassembles (demodulates) the audio frequency from the carrier frequency (Figure 6–3).

The 72 to 76 MHz band was the initial allocation by the FCC for HATs used by individuals with hearing loss. This frequency region encompasses a bandwidth of 4 MHz (or 4000 kHz). To permit the use of different FM systems that did not interfere with one another, this frequency region was further subdivided by FM manufacturers into 10 wideband (400 kHz wide) or 40 narrowband (100 kHz wide) channels. However, the separation of those channels was increased further to minimize cross-channel interference by allowing the individual channels to be no more than 50 kHz wide. In general, there would be only one transmitter and one or more receivers. Suppose, however, that three students with hearing loss need to use their FM system in the same building, but in two different classes occurring at the same time (e.g., 2 in geography versus 1 in history). In order to prevent interference, the two FM systems will need to be set on different transmission channels. The geography students and their teacher's transmitter might be on channel A (e.g., 72.2 MHz), while the history student and her teacher might be

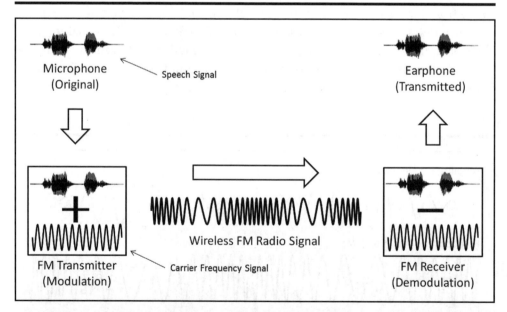

Figure 6–3. How FM systems work. The original speech signal is picked up by a microphone and sent to the FM transmitter to be combined (modulated) with the carrier frequency signal. Once modulated, the FM transmitter sends the FM signal wirelessly by radio to the FM receiver. The FM receiver will decompose (demodulate) the speech signal from the carrier frequency signal and send this to the earphone.

on channel D (73.4 MHz). In general, the same channel separation is applied for the newer 216 to 217 MHz frequency region, which the FCC later allocated. This frequency region has a bandwidth of 1 MHz (or 1,000 kHz), which was further subdivided into 20 (50 kHz wide) or 40 (25 kHz wide) bands. The 216 to 217 MHz frequency region appears to offer a slight improvement in reception and can be incorporated into smaller, ear-level FM receivers compared to the 72 to 76 MHz frequency region, though both are still routinely used today. Although there are both wide- and narrowband subdivision of channels, neither is more advantageous than the other. In addition, neither of the two frequency regions nor their two bandwidth distinctions is fully free from interference.

Applications of FM Technology

The perceived benefit of an FM system is the fact that the speech signal can be transmitted over long distances, against background noise, and through walls to be delivered directly into a student's (or patron's) ear. From Chapter 3, we know that as sound travels, it will lose energy over distance and often mixes with background noise. Counteracting these two issues is a way of improving the signal-to-noise ratio (SNR). It is desirable that the speech signal always be louder than the noise (a positive dB value), and a +10 dB SNR should be an easier listening situation compared to a +2 dB SNR. Illus-

trated visually in Figure 6–4, as distance increases from the original signal with background noise without an FM system, the SNR decreases from +6 to +2 dB. With an FM system, however, the SNR remains steady at +10 dB irrespective of distance. Viewed another way, Figure 6–5 illustrates the loss of energy with distance in a classroom from 65 dB SPL at 3 feet down to 53 dB SPL (i.e., following the Inverse Square Law). With an FM system, the student in the back row would have the same access to sound as the students in the front row. A third issue, related to noise, is reverberation, which is when multiple copies of the original signal plus background noise combine and are reflected off the hard surfaces in a room. Cafeterias obviously have more reverberation than a small medical examination room, making it more difficult to understand speech in the cafeteria than the examination room. With this in mind, below are example applications of FM systems.

Personal FM Systems

Personal FM systems come in different packages. On the one hand, the product package may be purchased from a retailer or audiologist, complete with belt-worn microphone/transmitter and receiver units to be used with one or more of a variety of different coupling options (e.g., headphones, earbuds, induction neckloop, induction silhouette [earhook], or direct-audio input cable.) On the other hand, the product package may be ordered by an audiologist and customized

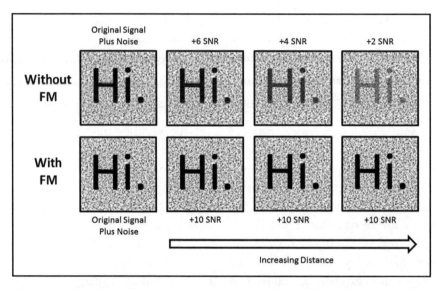

Figure 6–4. How FM systems provide improved signal-to-noise ratio (SNR). In each box is a gray shaded area to represent the background noise. The word "Hi." represents the speech signal of interest. From left to right, we can see the effect of increasing distance on SNR from the original source without the FM system. That is, the SNR decreases from +6 to +2 dB. This is represented visually with the word gradually fading into the noise. With the FM system, SNR remains constant at +10 dB regardless of increasing distance. This improvement (or maintenance) of SNR can also be seen with other hearing assistive technologies, such as induction loop systems and infrared (IR) systems.

in conjunction with personal hearing aids or implantable devices with an integrated (built-in) FM receiver or add-on FM receiver unit (audio shoe; Figure 6–6) to be used with a compatible microphone/transmitter (Figure 6–7). Regardless of the personal FM product package used, the fundamental operation is the same. The microphone/transmitter will be placed on the person who is speaking (e.g., teacher, parent, spouse, or friend) or it can be placed near a sound source of interest (e.g., next to a television/radio or on a podium). Unless there is only one frequency channel, the user will need to make sure that the microphone and receivers are "tuned" to each other by being on the same channel.

It may not be apparent at first, but it is important to understand the different coupling options with FM receiver units (unless an integrated FM or FM audio shoe is used). Figure 6–8 shows a number of different coupling options, with further description as follows: For individuals without hearing aids or implantable devices, a pair of headphones or earbuds will provide acoustic coupling, and users should be able to adjust the FM receiver volume control to optimize listening comfort.

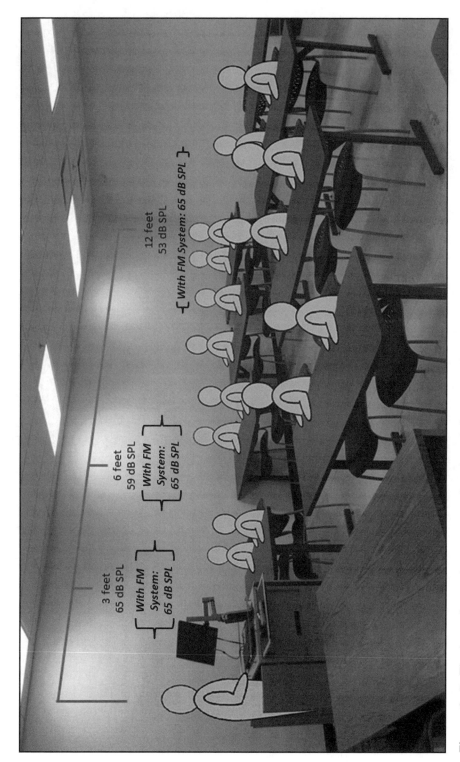

Figure 6–5. The loss of sound energy as a function of distance without an FM system. With an FM system, the speech signal is maintained at a constant level (65 dB SPL) such that the students in the back row have the same access as the students in the front row.

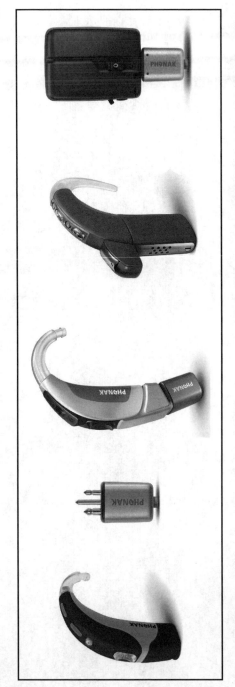

Figure 6–6. Examples of FM systems customized to work with various hearing aids and implantable devices. The hearing aid on the far left has an integrated FM receiver, whereas the remaining are a hearing aid, cochlear implant, and BAHA implant using a Phonak MLx-type audio shoe (*example MLx shown second from the left*). Images courtesy of Phonak.

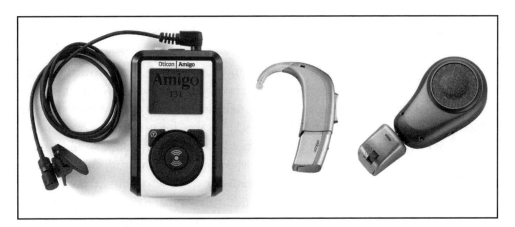

Figure 6–7. Example of an Oticon Amigo microphone/transmitter unit, hearing aid with Oticon R12 receiver, and Oticon Medical Ponto (bone-anchored) with Oticon R2BA receiver. Images courtesy of Oticon and Oticon Medical.

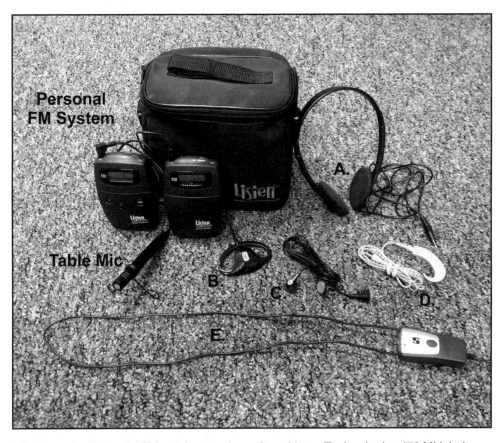

Figure 6–8. Example FM product package from Listen Technologies (72 MHz) shown with a variety of different coupling options. Coupling options are as follows: **A–E.** headphones, earphone, earbuds, induction silhouette (earhook), and induction neckloop (powered). Photo credit: Samuel R. Atcherson, PhD.

For individuals with telecoils built into their hearing aid or implantable device, there are a number of coupling options: induction neckloop or induction silhouette (earhook). Interestingly, these induction options produce signals only the telecoil user can hear. Many may not be aware, but headphones can be used as an induction coupling option as well, since, like induction neckloops and silhouettes, they are also capable of producing a small magnetic field around the headphone speakers (see Chapter 7). Last, for some hearing aids and implantable devices, there may be a direct-audio input coupling option that calls for the use of a cable. Here, the output of the FM receiver is introduced directly (i.e., hardwired) into the hearing aid or implantable device.

Personal FM systems are so versatile that additional benefits have been conceived and developed for them. For example, hearing aid company Phonak offers a family of FM transmitters that, through direct, hardwired connection, can transmit information from other electronic devices such as the television, MP3 players, and computers. The same transmitter can also be used by a teacher in a classroom, by a parent in the car, and in the middle of a large conference room table.

Large Area FM Systems

For large areas, such as an auditorium or theater, an FM system that can be connected to an already existing public address (PA) system may be worthwhile. These large area systems come with a wall-mounted transmitter antenna, which can transmit FM signals over a longer range than for personal FM systems. Generally, multiple receiver units come with a large area kit using acoustic coupling headphones or earphones for individuals who do not have hearing aids. However, individuals with telecoils in their hearing aid or implantable device may be able to receive magnetic signals from the headphones. Alternatively, the FM receiver may be used with an induction neckloop or direct-audio input cable if one is provided and appropriate.

Another solution for large areas, such as classrooms and lecture halls, is an FM soundfield system. The teacher or lecturer would still use a microphone transmitter, but rather than a select number of people using FM receiver units, the entire room is filled acoustically with an amplified sound similar to a PA system. In this case, the soundfield (loudspeaker) system is the receiver, and all students in the room benefit from an improved SNR. Another benefit is reduced vocal strain and fatigue, better classroom management, and less stress for the teacher or lecturer. Figure 6–9 shows an example FM soundfield system.

Advantages and Disadvantages of FM Technology

It is to be expected that no HAT will serve all purposes in all situations with individuals of all ages. In terms of advantages, FM systems are easy to set up and use, whether for personal use or for public use. They can provide access to speech sounds and maintain a positive SNR. For

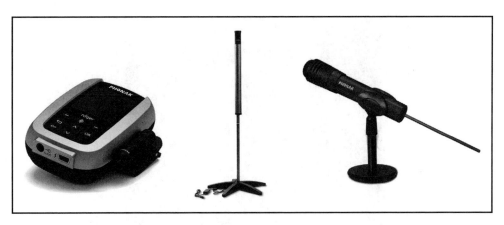

Figure 6–9. Example floor-style FM soundfield system (products not to scale). From left to right: Phonak Inspiro microphone transmitter; Phonak DigiMaster receiver and loudspeaker; and Phonak DymaMic microphone transmitter. The Inspiro is used by the teacher or lecturer, whereas the DynaMic is a pass-around microphone used by the class or meeting participants for comments and questions. The DigiMaster loudspeaker stands several feet high (or can be wall mounted). Images courtesy of Phonak.

personal FM systems, there are a variety of ways in which a microphone/transmitter can be used for education, communication, and entertainment. Disadvantages include some potential radio frequency interference by other non-FM systems, interference from other FM systems on the same or adjacent channels, compatibility issues with other FM products, coupling issues with public FM receivers, and the need to carry FM receivers around. Nevertheless, the benefits of FM often outweigh the disadvantages.

alert customers that they are available. There are several places to purchase or download these signs to post on walls, windows, and digital or print communications. The logo for induction loop systems is based on the International Symbol for Hearing Loss and has an ear with a line drawn through it (to signify hearing loss) (Figure 6–10). More information about the logo can be found on the Center for Hearing Loss Help (http://www.hear inglosshelp.com) and the Hearing Loop (http://www.hearingloop.org) websites.

Public Signage

For public areas offering HAT for use, signs should be posted with the International Symbol for Hearing Loss to

From Fixed to Dynamic/ Adaptive FM

With FM systems, it is possible to reach SNRs of 20 dB or greater. When FM is

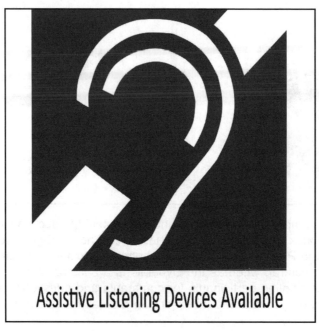

Figure 6–10. Sign with the International Symbol for Hearing Loss suitable for use to advertise available FM receivers.

combined with hearing aids, a common recommendation is to electroacoustically verify that the FM output is 10 dB greater or higher than the hearing aid output. The way this +10 dB advantage is achieved is with the understanding that speech picked up by the hearing aid alone would vary between 60 and 70 dB SPL (typical of conversation speech), whereas the speech picked up by an FM microphone/transmitter would vary between 70 and 80 dB SPL. Such SNR advantage is useful to counteract the effects of distance and noise. However, using a fixed +10 dB advantage in FM systems assumes that the noise will never change and that the SNR setting should never change. This "fixed"

+10 dB SNR approach is a limitation of many traditional FM systems. Recently, dynamic/adaptive FM systems have been designed to overcome the fixed, traditional FM issue. Dynamic/adaptive FM systems use sophisticated algorithms to enhance speech in varying noise levels and changing distance. In both hearing aid and cochlear implant users, dynamic/adaptive FM has been shown to be far superior to traditional FM systems, especially when noise levels increase (Thibodeau, 2014; Wolfe et al., 2009). Figure 6–11 illustrates how dynamic/adaptive FM compares to the traditional FM with both hearing aids and cochlear implants as a function of increasing back-

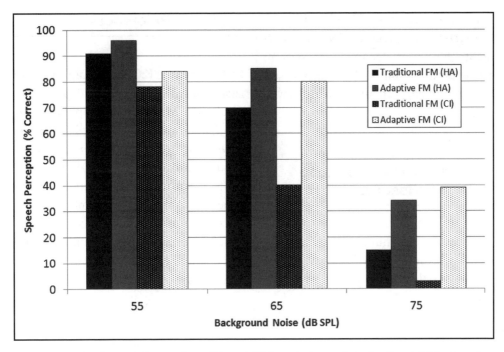

Figure 6–11. Comparison of traditional FM and dynamic/adaptive FM in hearing aid and cochlear implant users on speech perception performance as a function of increasing background noise levels. These data were extracted and combined from Wolfe et al. (2009) and Thibodeau (2014).

ground noise levels. Notice that as noise levels increase from 55 to 75 dB, overall speech perception performance declines. However, it should also be observed that as noise increases, the dynamic/adaptive FM consistently outperforms the traditional FM.

Summary

FM systems are a powerful and versatile HAT using radio frequency transmission to help counteract the effect of distance and noise. A side benefit is that the individual using the microphone/transmitter can minimize vocal fatigue over the course of a long day of speaking. FM systems can be used for communication, education, and entertainment. With FM, speech sounds and other signals of interest can be wirelessly transmitted to a listeners' ears via hearing aids with integrated FM, using FM audio shoes with hearing aids and implantable devices, or via one of several coupling options such as acoustic headphones and induction neckloops. FM transmission has also been useful in large area soundfield loudspeaker systems. Finally, although FM systems are great for SNR improvement, the newer dynamic FM systems are rendering traditional (fixed) FM systems as limited, particularly in high levels of noise.

Selected Audio-Video Resources

- Personal FM Simulation: http://www.youtube.com/watch?v=1l37lzLIgQU

References

Thibodeau, L. (2014). Comparison of speech recognition with adaptive digital and FM remote microphone hearing assistance technology by listeners who use hearing aids. *American Journal of Audiology, 23*(2), 201–210.

Wolfe, J., Schafer, E. C., Heldner, B., Mülder, H., Ward, E., & Vincent, B. (2009). Evaluation of speech recognition in noise with cochlear implants and dynamic FM. *Journal of the American Academy of Audiology, 20*(7), 409–421.

7

Induction and Hearing Loop Systems

Overview

The use of induction is one of the most underused of the various hearing assistive technologies (HATs), at least here in the United States. Professionals, educators, public venue personnel, and consumers seem to be more familiar with HATs that are a pair of headsets and accompanying receiver unit, or are a part of an accommodation in a school (e.g., frequency-modulated [FM] system [Chapter 6] or infrared [IR] system [Chapter 8]). In the case of schoolchildren, there may be a wearable device or an add-on to the child's hearing aids or implant device that allows

better reception of the teacher's voice and potentially access to other students' voices in the classroom. While these are wonderful, wireless technologies that serve their purpose with important advantages, it is the inexpensively manufactured and cost-effective induction hearing loop technology that unfortunately has either been largely forgotten, or its significance downplayed. Currently, there is renewed interest and awareness with individual advocacy efforts by hearing professionals and consumers alike, and with the large-scale "Get in the Hearing Loop" campaign (http://www.hearingloss.org/content/get-hearing-loop) and the International Hearing Loop conferences (http://www.hearinglink.org/loop-conference). In this chapter, we describe the components of induction, beginning with a telecoil.

What Is a Telecoil?

The telecoil (also called a T-coil) is the most important component of induction technology. A telecoil is made up of a small metal rod encircled many times by thin copper wire (looking like a tiny spool of thread). Telecoils are quite small (Figure 7–1), and they are easily built into hearing aids and implantable hearing devices (Figures 7–2 and 7–3). Telecoils are receivers and behave similarly to a microphone. Conventional microphones detect sounds in the form of acoustic air-pressure changes, and they convert these changes to an alternating electric current. Telecoils, on the other hand, detect magnetic field changes. When telecoils encounter a magnetic field that changes over time, an alternating electric current is generated in the "coil" of wire. This action is referred to as "induction," from which we have concepts such as induction coils (telecoil) and induction loops. Electromagnetism is a complex, technical topic that can be described in many different forms. In its simplest form, when an ordinary magnet is allowed to move back and forth within a coil of wire, electric current will move back and forth in the coil of wire. The magnet, in this case,

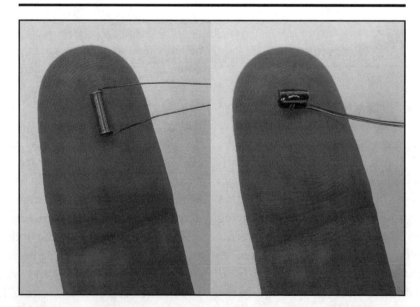

Figure 7–1. Examples of telecoils on the end of an adult finger. On the left is a passive telecoil and on the right is an amplified telecoil. Images courtesy of Jason A. Galster, PhD of Galster.net.

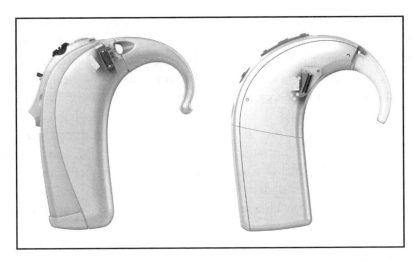

Figure 7–2. Illustrative (cutaway) examples of the telecoil within the casing of two generations of cochlear implant processors (headpiece and cable not shown). Images courtesy of Advanced Bionics.

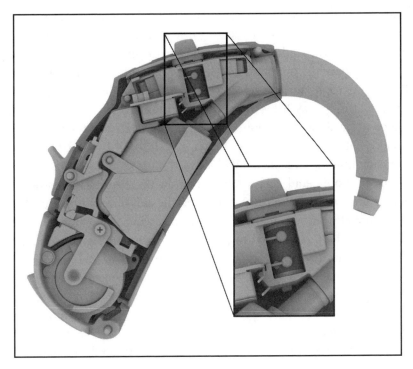

Figure 7–3. Illustrative example of telecoil (*see enlarged image*) in a behind-the-ear hearing aid with right side of the case open. Image courtesy of Phonak.

is the energy source. Conversely, when another energy source forces current back and forth through a coil of wire, the coil of wire will produce a magnetic field. With a small telecoil, the energy of the magnetic field can be harnessed, amplified, and processed by a hearing aid or implant device. Figure 7–4 illustrates the basic pathway through which a telecoil harnesses a magnetic audio signal to be amplified and delivered through a small loudspeaker.

Although not always common knowledge, telephones (including many mobile phones) and portable music headphones produce both acoustic and magnetic signals. The diaphragm of the loudspeaker produces the acoustic signal; the magnet and coil of wire behind the diaphragm produce a concurrent magnetic field. Some hearing aid or implant device users may have the option of having both the microphone and telecoil activated so that they may listen on the telephone or to music with headphones (magnetically) while also being able to hear their surroundings (acoustically). As described in more detail below, telecoils can be paired with a behind-the-ear induction silhouette or personal neckloop or to a room loop connected to an electronic sound source (e.g., television or any public address–type system at a place of worship, theater, or transportation vehicle).

Every hearing aid and implant device is different, but if there is sufficient space, a telecoil can be added upon purchase, or it can be built in as one of several features. If there is a telecoil, its physical orienta-

tion is hearing device specific. Some hearing devices have a manual toggle switch. Years ago, toggle switches were quite common on analog hearing aids with plainly marked labels: "M" for microphone, "T" for telephone (or telecoil), and "O" for off. Sometimes, instead of "T" they were marked "MT" for microphone and telephone (telecoil). In this chapter, we describe various real-life situations and use the terms MT mode and T mode to illustrate the various uses. In modern day hearing aids, those labels are generally no longer present, and are now buried within other types of button or lever switches that cycle through two or more programs, or they are activated using a handheld program remote control. In consultation with the hearing instrument professional, the various programs could be set up in the software to cycle with every button press, for example, through quiet environments (program 1), noisy environments (program 2), music (program 3), telecoil (program 4), and back again. Telecoils must be manually activated in order to use them with a variety of induction hearing loop products. Some hearing aids have automatic telecoils that activate when a telephone receiver with a strong magnetic signal is placed next to the hearing aid. If the magnetic signal is weak, a small magnet with adhesive on one side can be added to the telephone receiver to help the automatic telecoil activate. It should be noted that automatic telecoils are generally not effective for use with induction hearing loop products.

We are generally not accustomed to thinking about sound in magnetic form.

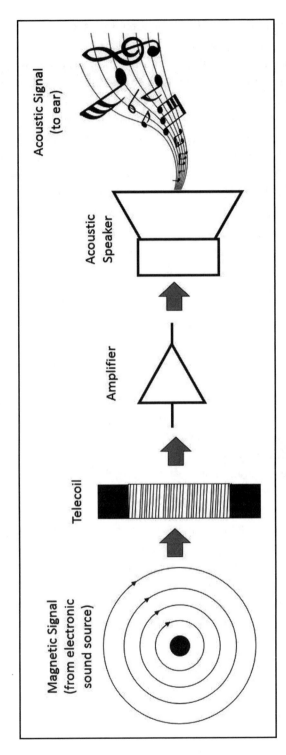

Figure 7–4. Simplified illustration of an induction pathway. The telecoil picks up the magnetic signal from an electronic sound source, which is then amplified and converted from an electric to acoustic signal. The magnetic signal shown here is represented by the magnetic flux lines moving concentrically in a perpendicular manner around the cross-sectional cut of the loop wire (*black circle*). See also Figure 7–5.

Herein lies the beauty of induction technology. When there is a personal telecoil and an induction system, the hearing aid or implant device user can discretely and wirelessly pick up sound without the use of additional devices such as FM or IR technology. This experience has been described as "doubling the functionality of hearing aids" (Myers, 2010) and "telecoils act as mini loudspeakers" (Greenemeier, 2009). Myers has also described this experience as having "an Internet Wi-Fi hotspot." Just as laptops and smartphones can connect to wireless Internet networks, a telecoil can connect to induction systems wirelessly. The real benefit of telecoils with induction systems is an improvement of signal-to-noise ratio (SNR) (see Chapter 3). To illustrate the dual functionality of hearing aids (and implant devices), Figure 7–5 shows spectrograms of a pair of audio recordings, one with the telecoil turned on (lower photo) and one turned off (upper photo), while inside a highly reverberant place of worship with an installed induction loop system. Reverberation has the effect of causing sounds to bounce all over the walls, floor, and ceilings to the point that speech sounds are smeared together. With the telecoil turned on (and microphone turned off), the reverberation is drastically reduced and the speech sounds are clearer. Readers are encouraged to listen to the difference using the following Internet link: https://www.youtube.com/watch?v=_3XoVrUjfaY.

Avid users of telecoils will attest that there can be a "sweet spot" when using telecoils with induction systems. This phenomenon is due to the physical shape and orientation of a telecoil, which affects its ability to pick up the magnetic signal. As a purely illustrative example, an audio induction loop around a room is positioned horizontally, while the magnetic field radiates from the loop in a vertical manner toward the center of the room (perpendicular to the flow of electric current through the wire). The magnetic field produces what are called flux lines, and within a loop, the flux lines radiate, delivering time-varying magnetic signals. To best harness the magnetic signal coming from the loop, the telecoil must be oriented properly with respect to the flux lines. Increasing the signal strength and overall loudness. Figure 7–6 shows examples of optimal, acceptable, and poor physical orientation of the telecoil to the flux lines. Some telecoils may need to be boosted by the hearing professional, if they appear to be weak (see the section entitled Telecoil Programming and Verification by Hearing Professionals later in this chapter).

There is a word of caution, however. Some hearing aids are equipped with an automatic telecoil, such as for use with telephones. The idea here is that when a telephone is placed against the hearing aid, the telecoil will automatically activate. This setup works if the hearing aid has the proper electronic component to detect a strong magnetic field. This electronic component may have several names, but it is a magnetic reed switch or a giant magnetoresistor (GMR). Some telephones may not have a strong enough magnetic field to activate the telecoil. In

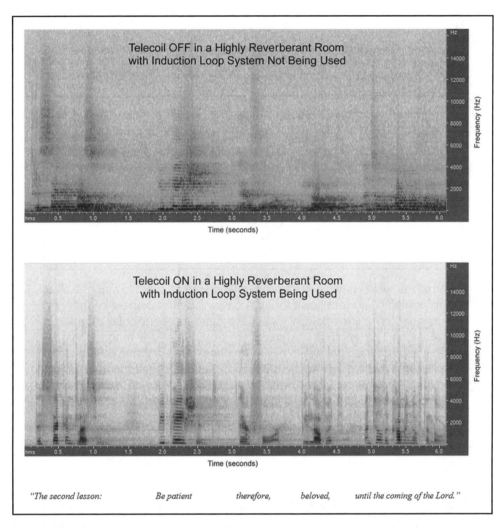

Figure 7–5. Spectrograms of a pair of audio recordings in a highly reverberant place of worship with installed induction loop system. Spectrograms show speech energy and frequency over time (*the blackened areas*). When the telecoil is off (*top trace*), the spectrogram shows a smearing effect of speech sounds, and the dark gray background illustrates the background noise level. When the telecoil is turned on (microphone off), the detail of speech sounds is much more apparent and the lighter gray background shows a reduction in the background noise. Audio recordings courtesy of Richard Einhorn, Juliëtte Sterkens, AuD, and LeRoy "Max" Maxfield.

this case, stick-on magnets can be added to the telephone headset to improve the likelihood that the GMR will activate the telecoil. These stick-on magnets are available from various hearing aid manufacturers.

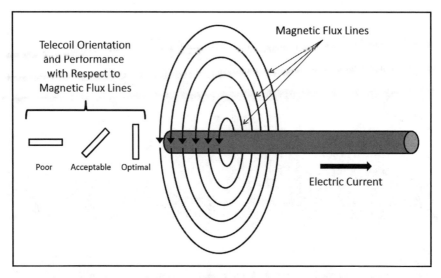

Figure 7–6. Importance of telecoil orientation with respect to magnetic flux lines. As electric current flows through a wire loop in a horizontal manner, the magnetic flux lines flow in a concentric and perpendicular manner to the wire loop. The length of the telecoil will best receive the magnetic signal when it is positioned parallel to the magnetic flux lines. When the telecoil's orientation is displaced from the parallel position to the magnetic flux lines, the signal strength will decrease. Many telecoils are preoriented in the hearing aid or implant device. However, the user may have to reposition his or her head, headphone, or phone (or other induction device) to find the "sweet spot" where the signal is optimized.

Applications of Induction Technology

We now appreciate that the telecoil, as a receiver, is the most important component in induction technology. What signals would we want to capture? Ideally, the signal would be anything we want to hear. This may be a teacher in a classroom, a lecturer in a workshop, any speaker in a house of worship, stage participants in a theater, music at a symphony orchestra, sports announcer at a live sporting event, television show, driver or tour guide in a bus, gate announcers at an airport, or music or books from a digital device. How we get that magnetic signal to the telecoil can come in many forms involving small, wearable devices that are placed right next to the hearing aid or implant device or wire-based loops that cover a large listening area.

Signs should be posted with the International Symbol for Hearing Loss to alert customers and that an induction loop system, or other HAT, is available. There are several places to purchase or download these signs to post on walls, windows, and digital or print communications. The logo for induction loop systems is based on the

International Symbol for Hearing Loss and has an ear with a line drawn through it (to signify hearing loss) and a capital "T" (to signify telecoil) in the bottom right-hand corner (Figure 7–7). More information about the logo can be found on the Center for Hearing Loss Help (http://www.hearinglosshelp.com) and the Hearing Loop (http://www.hearingloop.org) websites.

In the sections below, the application of telecoils with a wide variety of induction methods is discussed. We begin our discussion with induction loop systems first as another wireless HAT (compare to FM systems in Chapter 6 and infrared systems in Chapter 8). From there, we introduce additional devices and situations when telecoils and induction technology may also be beneficial.

Room or Large Area Hearing Loop Systems

Installation of induction loop systems will depend on the purpose, location, and

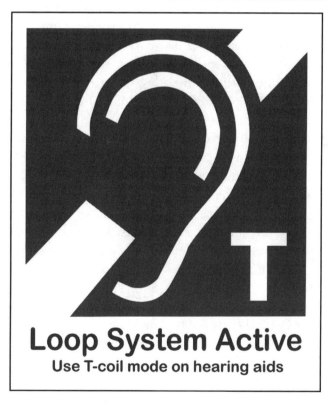

Figure 7–7. Example of hearing loop logo with instructions at the bottom to activate telecoil. If induction loop receivers are available, additional instructions or a second sign (or communication) will be required. Image courtesy of Neil Bauman, PhD, of Center for Hearing Loss Help.

skill level of the installer. There are quite a few residential installation packages that cost $100 to $300, which can be installed quite easily by the consumer with a little planning, comfort with connecting electronics, and typical household tools. These small residential kits are perfect for living rooms and bedrooms, and they have installation instruction manuals. Figure 7–8 shows the basic components and the relative ease of installation of a residential induction loop system kit with a small amplifier box, power supply, ~100 feet of 20- to 22-gauge wire to loop a room, and red and white audio cables to connect to a television. Some of these residential installation kits may offer a small microphone port that could be used for a small public address system. For these small residential loop systems, the installer should minimize trips and falls by securing the wire loop to the intersection of the floor and wall, or taping it down underneath the bed, couch, carpet, or rug. Although not as common, the loop could be elevated to the intersection of the ceiling and wall or be hidden above acoustic tiling. To maximize the magnetic signal, the wire loop should be above or below head level. Residential loop system users should be aware that individuals on floors above or below the loop may also be able to "listen in" with their telecoils. If the individual with hearing loss does not have his or her own hearing aids or implants with telecoil, a portable induction loop receiver can be purchased and used with a standard pair of headphones or earphones.

Induction loop systems for larger public and commercial areas such as meeting rooms, places of worship, theaters, lecture halls, auditoriums, sports arenas, and performing arts venues may cost anywhere from $1,000 to upwards of $150,000. The cost will depend on the size and construction of the room and whether the installation will be in a new facility or in one that requires retrofitting to bury the wire loop into the structure. Generally speaking, installation for a preplanned new facility, or one that is already being remodeled, will be cheaper than retrofitting. These installations will require professionals who are specially trained to connect the loop system to existing audio systems, while minimizing electromagnetic interference (EMI) and maximizing the capabilities of the loop system. These goals are met by conforming to IEC60118-4 (International Electrotechnical Commission, 2006), which specifies the frequency response, field strength, background noise, and various subjective tests. The IEC standard provides an average reference of 100 milliamps per meter (or 100 mA/m) with a peak output of 400 mA/m. What this means is that when a loop system can produce an average output of 100 mA/m, then the acoustic equivalent is about 70 dB SPL. These values are important in the selection, programming, and verification of telecoils in hearing aids. In very large rooms, there will often be more than one loop and more than one amplifier. Furthermore, the individual loops may be placed into patterns that preserve sound quality while minimizing "null zones" or "dead spots." For example, if there are several fixed rows of seats, a single wire can be "figure-8" looped around each row.

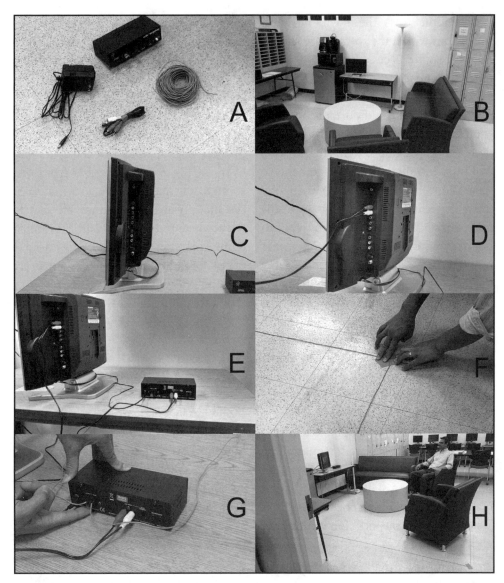

Figure 7–8. Example of residential induction loop system. **A.** Basic components of the kit. **B.** Room/area to have induction loop system installed. **C.** Locating red and white audio outputs on the back/side of the television. **D.** Plugging in the red and white audio cables to the television audio outputs. **E.** Connecting the other end of the audio cables into the loop amplifier red and white audio inputs. **F.** Looping the room/area with the wire and securing it (clips, hooks, tape, etc.). **G.** Connecting the wire loop to the back of the loop amplifier. **H.** Enjoying the fruits of our labor after activating the telecoil (user in this figure wears a cochlear implant with programmable telecoil) and adjusting the television and loop amplifier to volume preferences. Photo credit: Clifford A. Franklin, PhD.

Between the rows there will be "null zones," but within the rows, there should be good sound access. Figure 7–9 illustrates a comparison between a common perimeter room loop and a "movie-style" single array loop. An important consideration for these professionals is the installation of multiple loop systems in the same building. Installers will work to achieve separation of different loops systems by using cancellation loop arrays to minimize energy "spill" or "bleedover" into one or more adjacent rooms. Ampetronic Limited has an excellent resource for the design of induction loop systems for those interested (http://www.ampetronic .com/Designing-induction-loops).

Finally, induction loop systems can be installed in vehicles (e.g., cars and boats) or other forms of public or private transportation (e.g., taxi, subway, ferry, and bus). These loop systems would enable the driver or tour guide to speak into a microphone and the loop system would allow the telecoil user to benefit. Obviously, the skill level of the installer will need to be higher in order to install one of these loop systems into a transportation vehicle.

Advantages and Disadvantages of Room or Large Area Hearing Loop Systems

It is to be expected that no HAT will serve all purposes in all situations with individuals of all ages. The most obvious advantage of induction technology is the portability of telecoils, which can be built directly into hearing aids and implant devices. In addition, induction loop systems are generally low cost and

easy to maintain compared to other assistive listening technologies. The disadvantages, however, involve the susceptibility of the telecoil to a variety of factors that reduce sound quality. For example, EMI, other electric devices (e.g., fluorescent lighting), power line hums, poor telecoil-to-loop magnetic flux orientation, "spillover" of the magnetic signal from one room to an adjacent room, and increased distance from the loop may all lead to reduced sound quality and audibility. Some induction loop systems are portable (a possible advantage), whereas others are permanently installed into the room or structure (a possible disadvantage).

Short Range and Portable Loops

Induction loop systems for rooms, public areas, and transportation are all wonderful, but they are not suitable for all situations. It may not be necessary to loop an entire room or space when one might get by with a personal loop. A clever loop system is one in the form of a thin pad that can be placed on a chair or under a seat cushion (Figure 7–10). With a loop pad, the loop wires are organized within a flat, fabric-like accessory that can be connected to an audio loop amplifier. The audio loop amplifier is then connected to anything the telecoil user wants to gain better access to, such as a television, music player, or even a microphone strategically placed in a room or car. The loop pad has a short range of only a few feet, and it will benefit only one or two people sitting directly on top of it. Because the

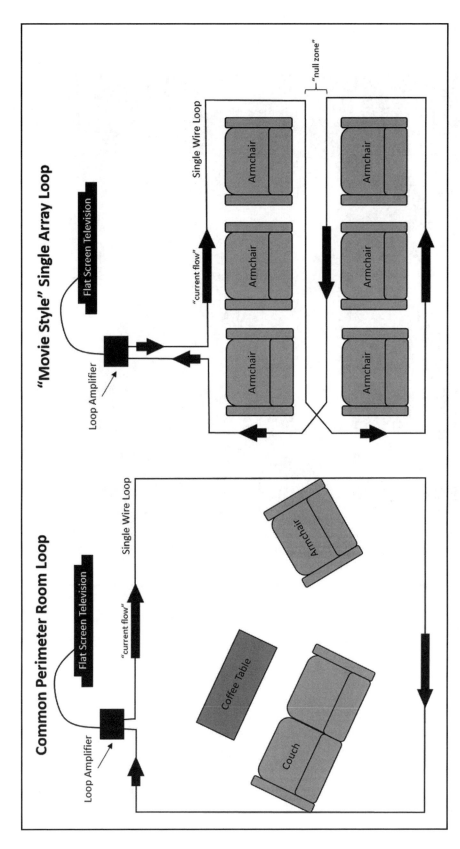

Figure 7–9. Examples of wire arrays in perimeter loop (*left*) and single array loop (*right*) with a single loop amplifier. While both scenarios use a single loop wire, the single array loop is arranged to form smaller looped areas using a "figure-8" pattern with established "null zone" areas in fixed seating arrangements found in movie theaters or lecture halls.

121

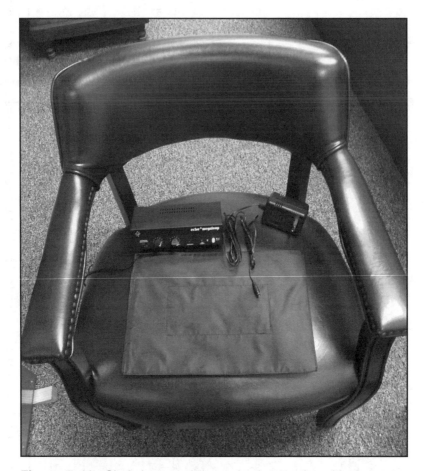

Figure 7–10. Chair loop pad example that works with the same induction loop system setup shown in Figure 7–8. Photo credit: Samuel R. Atcherson, PhD.

loop pad "loop" is not built into the floor, wall, or ceiling, it is portable and can be taken for use elsewhere.

Another short-range solution involves situations where a person needs to hear a bank teller or cashier. Here, a private, one-on-one induction loop is needed rather than a public induction loop. There are a few products that would serve this purpose and are designed to create short-range, countertop-style "hotspots" for the customer. Figure 7–11 shows two products that are portable, if they ever need to be moved to another location or used in a private consultation. Figure 7–12 shows another product that has more permanence but functions just like a countertop, portable system. A separate microphone is required (unless one is already built in to the device).

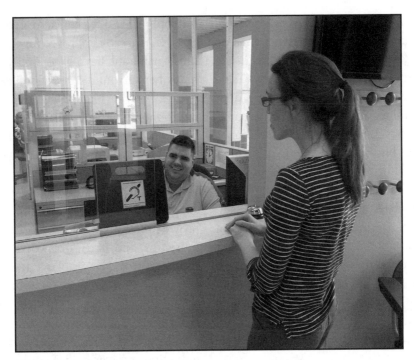

Figure 7–11. Example of short-range, countertop-style induction loop system with built-in microphone for use in one-on-one, over-the-counter situations. A telecoil activated within 3 to 5 feet of the countertop unit will be able to pick up the loop signal. Note that the induction loop logo is already prominently displayed on the counter-top unit. Photo credit: Samuel R. Atcherson, PhD.

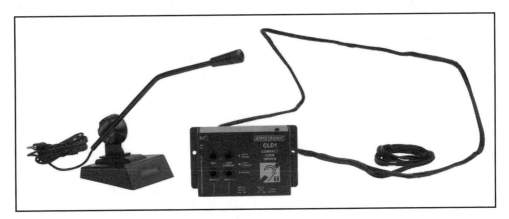

Figure 7–12. Another example of a short-range induction loop system for use in one-on-one situations, similar to the products in Figure 7–11. This product is not intended to be portable. Image courtesy of Listen Technologies.

Finally, there are several types of audio communication systems that do not fit the above scenarios such as drive-thru intercoms, ATM machines (automatic teller machines for banking), door entry intercoms, elevator lift intercoms, emergency/refuge help point intercoms, and taxi, bus, or transit system intercoms. These audio systems could be built (or retrofitted) with short-range loop systems to allow telecoil users to obtain access to broadcasted messages whether or not there is another speaker on the other end or if the message is already scripted. Again, the benefit here for the telecoil user is to improve the SNR, especially in noisy public areas. These systems will likely need to be professionally installed.

Ear- and Neck-Level Induction Devices

Nearly every headphone has the capacity to deliver both an acoustic and a magnetic signal by the design of the small loudspeakers built into them to deliver sound. When available, telecoil users can choose to use their microphone-only, microphone and telecoil, or telecoil-only modes depending on the situation and environment they are in. For example, if the intent is simply to enjoy music or video from a digital media player while in the quiet and comfort of one's home, the telecoil may be activated on its own and all other sources of environmental background noise would be cut out (T mode). In another scenario, the listener may choose to use headphones with both the microphone and telecoil activated so that the SNR is greatly improved for the digital music while still having the ability to hear his or her surroundings. A good example is on a noisy airplane. Keeping both the microphone and telecoil activated (MT mode) would simultaneously allow one to stay alert for intercom messages from the pilot or stewards, while watching an in-flight movie. Headphones may also be supplied with FM and infrared systems provided in public venues (e.g., theaters, museums, and houses of worship), and the hearing aid or implant device user should still be able to take advantage of induction between the telecoil and headphone. For those who do not have a built-in hearing aid telecoil, a separate induction receiver device could be used with a pair of ordinary headphones.

Options other than bulky headphones include personal induction neckloops and behind-the-ear induction silhouettes. Neckloops are not unlike room loops, except that the listener's head is now looped. Silhouettes got their name because they were made initially to look like hearing aids and be placed on the ear between the hearing aid and the head. Inside these induction silhouettes is a coil loop that will produce a magnetic field from the current that passes through it from the electronic sound device. Anecdotally, induction silhouettes are often thought to be more effective than neck loops because of the closer proximity to the telecoil and because they do not require much volume control amplification. However, some neckloops are powered to provide additional gain. All of these ear- and neck-level devices and possible options for use are shown in Figure 7–13.

Landline and Mobile Phones

Some landline and mobile phones may be compatible with telecoils. Landline phones that are hearing aid compatible (HAC) should be readily available, given the existence of the U.S. Hearing Aid Compatibility Act of 1989. Mobile phones, on the other hand, have lagged behind their landline counterparts because public mobile and wireless phones were exempt from the Act until 2003. In 2003, the Federal Communications Commission (FCC) determined that the exemption for mobile and wireless phones would severely limit accessibility for individuals with hearing loss. Because of this determination, the FCC began establishing rules for hearing aid compatibility for digital wireless phones. FCC regulations have since been tweaked with mandates that mobile phone providers carry a certain number of hearing aid compatible mobile phones and/or some minimum quality/rating of hearing aid compatibility under test standards. Briefly, many mobile phones will have M (microphone) or T (telecoil) ratings to permit acoustic and/or inductive coupling. For inductive coupling, a

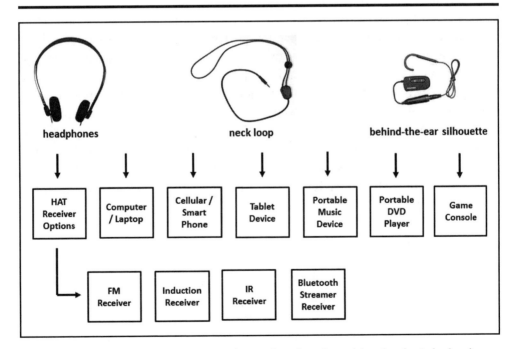

Figure 7–13. Example of listener options when hearing aid or implant device has a built-in telecoil.

rating of T3 or T4 is best, which should have the least amount of interference. Readers should consult Chapter 11 for more in-depth information on telecommunications access, including the use of telecoils.

Telecoil Programming and Verification by Hearing Professionals

This section is directed primarily to hearing professionals, but the information will likely also be useful to consumers. As stated earlier, telecoils can be added to many hearing aids and implant devices to double their functionality. However, telecoils may need to be programmed and verified. With hearing aids, the telecoils (like microphones) are verified using a hearing aid test box that shows exactly what the hearing aid produces (amplitude frequency response) when a known signal is presented to it. The most recent standard at the time of this publication for assessing telecoils with a hearing aid test box is ANSI 3.22-2003 (American National Standards Institute, 2003). In ANSI 2003, there are two telecoil tests described: one for telephone simulation and one for loop simulation. Specifically, the hearing aid test box is capable of generating a magnetic field either inside the test box, or with an external accessory.

The ANSI 2003 standard contains a number of different abbreviations pertaining to the telecoil tests such as SPLITS (sound pressure level inductive telephone simulation), SPLIV (sound pressure level inductive vertical field), RSETS (relative simulation equivalent telephone sensitivity), and RTLS (relative test loop sensitivity) (Figure 7–14). As you might expect, SPLITS and RSETS go together, while SPLIV and RTLS go together. Here's how this works: The programmed hearing aid must first be measured in order to determine what the microphone amplitude frequency response is (specifically to obtain the reference test gain, RTG). Next, the telecoil is activated to conduct the two simulated tests. For the telephone simulation, the hearing aid is placed flush against the magnetic field simulator either in the box or external accessory and an amplitude frequency response is measured. For the loop simulation, the hearing aid is positioned vertically (as if it were on someone's ear) and a third amplitude frequency response is measured. From these two tests, the high-frequency average (HFA) SPLITS and SPLIV is calculated, and the RSETS and RTLS are calculated relative to the RTG for the microphone. If the RSETS and/or RTLS value is 0, then they are equivalent to the RTG, which is desirable. If the RSETS and/or RTLS have a negative value, it implies that the gain offered via the telecoil is less than that offered by the microphone, which is undesirable. Illustrative examples for the undesirable and desirable measurements are shown in Figure 7–15. Here, the hearing professional has the opportunity (if possible) to increase the gain for the telecoil so that it closely matches the gain for the microphone. It should be noted that despite equivalent telecoil and microphone response measured in a coupler,

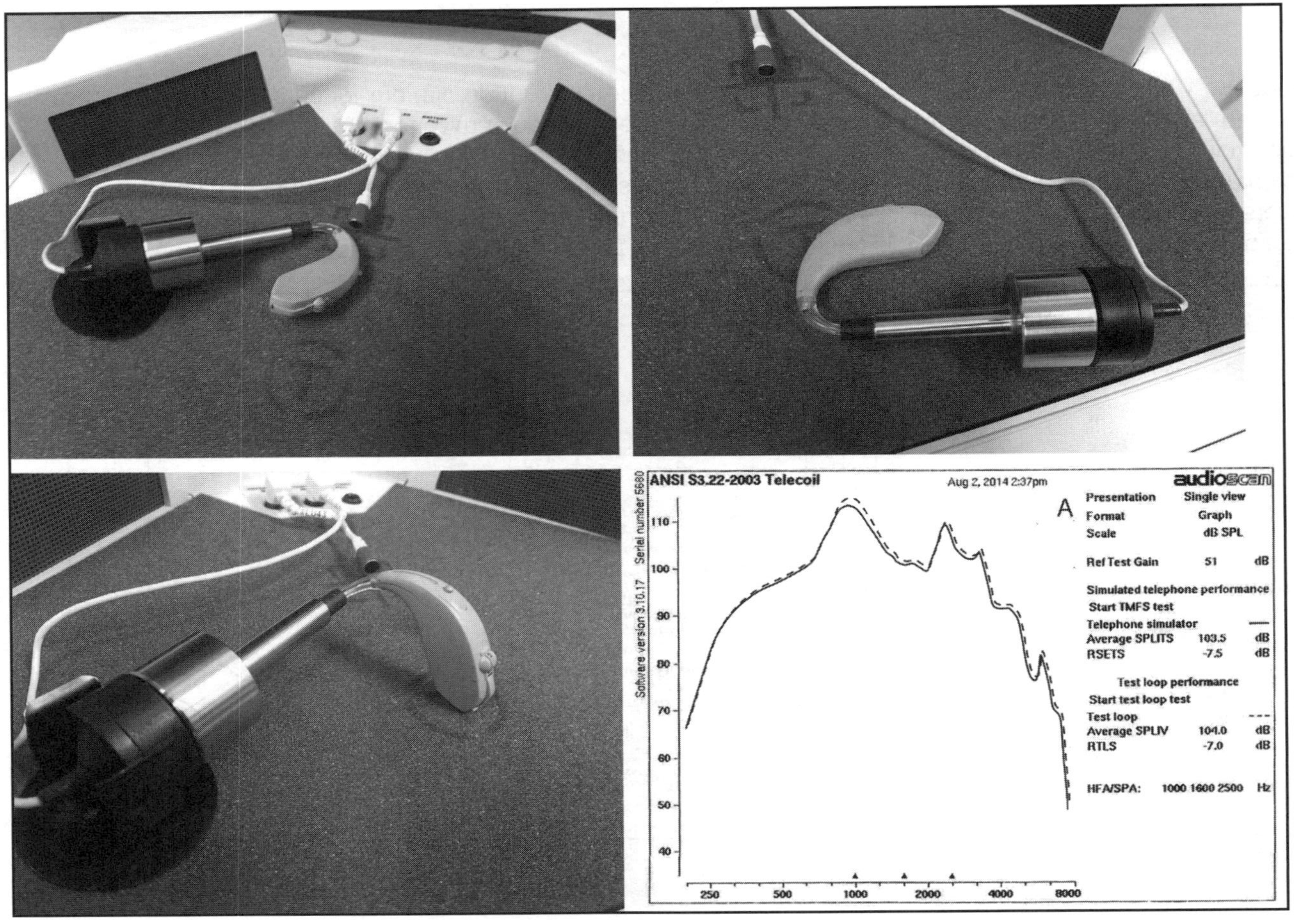

Figure 7–14. Using the Audioscan Verifit hearing aid test system, the microphone amplitude frequency response is first obtained at user settings in a 2-cc coupler (*top left*). Next, the hearing aid is switched to telecoil mode and is positioned on its side near the marked "T circle" for the telephone simulator test (*top right*). Finally, the hearing aid is positioned upright over the "T circle" for the loop simulator test (*bottom left*). At the conclusion of all tests, the RTG, SPLITS, RSETS, SPLIV, and RTLS values will be displayed. The RSETS and RTLS values suggest that the telecoil gain is between 7.0 and 7.5 dB less than the RTG (the microphone gain). Photo credit: Samuel R. Atcherson, PhD.

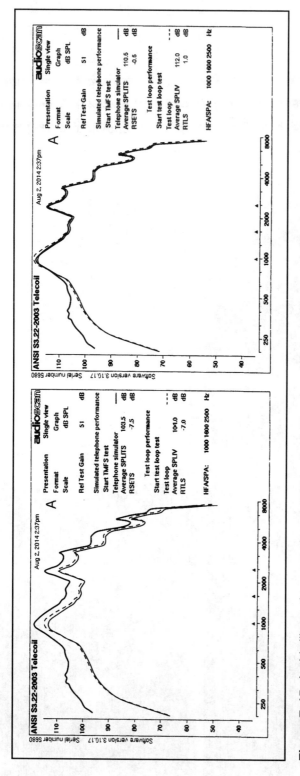

Figure 7–15. In this illustrative case, the printout on the left was modified to combine the RTG amplitude frequency response curve (*thick line*) from Figure 7–14 for comparison with the telephone (*thin line*) and loop (*dashed line*) simulator curves. Just glancing at the three curves in the printout on the left shows that the RTG curve is higher than the other two curves by about 7.5 and 7.0 dB for RSETS and RTLS, respectively. These suggest that the telecoil gain is underpowered. After increasing the telecoil gain, the RSETS and RTLS can be better matched to the RTG as shown in the printout on the right. Note that the gain for the telecoil is substantially less than for the microphone at frequencies below 1000 Hz. Photo credit: Samuel R. Atcherson, PhD.

Putterman and Valente (2012) reported that some patients may complain about less than satisfactory loudness with the telecoil. The reason for this lies in the difference in gain between the microphone and telecoil at frequencies below 1000 Hz. Specifically, the telecoil gain is lower than the microphone gain. These lower frequencies are where speech sounds derive their overall power (see right printout in Figure 7–15). To compensate, the telecoil gain may need to be increased so that the RSETS and/or RTLS reaches a positive value.

To ensure that hearing aids have good telecoils, hearing professionals should consult the hearing aid specification or datasheet and look for mention of telecoil or induction coil sensitivity and test loop sensitivity (TLS) values. Ideally, the TLS value should never be less than 0. As every specification or datasheet is different among manufacturers, alternatively, one can compare the output curves between the microphone RTG curve and telecoil curve. Be sure to look at the magnetic input signal before making the comparison between the RTG curve and the telecoil curve (i.e., 10 mA/m = 50 dB SPL, 31.6 mA/m = 60 dB SPL, and 100 mA/m = 70 dB SPL). For example, a hearing aid manufacturer may routinely test their telecoils at 10 mA/m. That input level is equivalent to 50 dB SPL, whereas RTG curves are routinely tested at 60 dB SPL giving the false impression that the telecoil is underpowered. Other hearing aid manufacturers will test the telecoil at 100 mA/m. A 100 mA/m input is equivalent to 70 dB SPL, will give the false impres-

sion that the telecoil is overpowered compared to the RTG at 60 dB SPL. The key is to make sure that the RTG and telecoil input levels are the same (31.6 mA/m = 60 dB SPL), or do a mental addition (10 mA/m versus 60 dB SPL) or subtraction (100 mA/m versus 60 dB SPL). Recall also that the IEC60118-4 standard specifies 100 mA/m as the average reference for the magnetic strength of an induction loop system with peaks up to 400 mA/m, which is useful for the telecoil's potential to work with induction loop systems.

Yanz and Pehringer (2003) offered seven steps to hearing professionals to standardize and optimize telecoils in hearing aids. We update these seven steps here: First, the hearing aid should have a telecoil (which may be passive or amplified). Second, the hearing aid should be programmable and have a dedicated program (memory) for the telecoil. Third, when appropriate, the hearing aid user may benefit from automatic switching between the microphone and telecoil for telephone use. (Remember that this will not be a good idea for induction loop systems.) Fourth, using a telephone with both hearing aids simultaneously is achievable today and may be considered in consultation with the hearing professional. Fifth, telecoils should be properly aligned for maximum benefit. Sixth, the telecoil should be optimized using a standard inductive signal source and test box as described above. Seventh, the user's home and workplace should be evaluated with a handheld field strength meter, available for purchase, and counseled accordingly.

Summary

In this chapter, much was covered about the versatility of a small, simple electronic component called a telecoil. A telecoil can double the functionality of hearing aids, and it is a cost-effective way to improve signal-to-noise ratio for both speech understanding and music enjoyment. Induction systems improve the quality of life for individuals with hearing loss in the home, workplace, and both private and public venues without the trouble of managing and maintaining other external devices. Consumers should consider taking greater advantage of telecoils and induction technology, and advocating for induction technology use in their communities. Hearing professionals can do their part by introducing this technology, increasing awareness, and becoming an advocate for the clients they serve.

Selected Print Resources

- http://www.audiology.org/ resources/consumer/ Documents/20101021_Telecoil_ factSheet.pdf
- http://www.hearingloss.org/ sites/default/files/docs/HLAA_ Telecoil_Brochure.pdf
- http://www.hearingloop.org
- http://www.loopamerica.com
- http://www.hearingloss.org/ content/get-hearing-loop

- http://www.scientificamerican .com/article/induction-hearing- loop/

Selected Audio-Video Resources

- Hearing Loop Demonstration: https://www.youtube.com/ watch?v=_3XoVrUjfaY
- Numerous Telecoil and Hearing Loop Videos from the Hearing Loss Association of America (HLAA): https://www.youtube .com/user/hearinglossaa

References

American National Standards Institute. (2003). *Specification of hearing aid characteristics* (ANSI S3.22-2003). Melville, NY.

Greenemeier, L. (2009, October 19). A loopy idea that works: Using telecoils to turn hearing aids into mini loudspeakers. *Scientific American*. Retrieved from http://www.scientific american.com/article/induction-hearing-loop/

International Electrotechnical Commission. (2006). *Electroacoustics—Hearing aids—Part 4: Induction loop systems for hearing aid purposes—Magnetic field strength*. Geneva, Switzerland.

Myers, D. G. (2010, February). Progress toward the looping of America—and doubled hearing aid functionality. *Hearing Review, 17*(2), 10–17.

Putterman, D. B., & Valente, M. (2012). Difference between the default telecoil (T-Coil) and programmed microphone frequency response in behind-the-ear (BTE) hearing aids. *Journal of the American Academy of Audiology, 23*(5), 366–378

Yanz, J. L., & Pehringer, J. (2003). Quantifying telecoil performance in the ear: Common practices and a new protocol. *Seminars in Hearing, 24*(1), 71–80.

8

Infrared (IR) Systems

Introduction

Infrared (IR) is a type of electromagnetic (EM) radiation with wavelengths of about 0.00001 meters (or 10^{-5} m). "Electromagnetic radiation" may sound frightening, but visible light is also on the EM radiation spectrum as *white light* with wavelengths of about 0.000001 meters (or 10^{-6} m). Humans cannot see IR transmissions with the unaided eye because the wavelengths are longer than those for visible light and are outside the range our eyes can detect. The visible spectrum of white light passing through the lenses of our eyes is what allows us to see the colors of the rainbow from red to violet. IR gets its name because it is below (infra-) the red portion of white light, but higher than radar, FM radio, television, and AM radio radiation. The difference between white light and IR is a good thing because it

provides a transmission pathway separate from humans' vision that has been made use of for assistive listening. There are two primary applications for IR technology for assisted listening: television and large meeting spaces (e.g., live theater and houses of worship). In this chapter we discuss each of these applications and show examples for each.

IR technology is based on light waves carrying a signal from one or more transmitters to one of several types of small, specialized receivers. Using television remote controls as an example, you may have noticed a small LED (light-emitting diode) bulb on the front, which is aimed toward the television. In some cases, the remote control has a black plastic window-like cover with an LED bulb just beneath. When the various buttons of the remote control are pressed, specific flashing light pulse patterns are sent to the television (or cable box). There are many conceivable light patterns that can be developed, but one way to think about this is in the form of binary digits (i.e., zeros and ones). For example, the zeros could be represented by a short light pulse, whereas a one could be represented by a long light pulse. An example pattern could look like 000 01001. The pulse pattern will contain information about which device the signal is to be directed to (e.g., television versus DVD player) and the command (e.g., volume up/down and channel up/down).

In the case of assistive listening devices, the information carried by sound is the signal to be sent from a transmitter to a receiver. The transmitter can convey sound from any one of many different audio devices and may also be used with a public address system. A technical description of exactly how IR technology works to transmit sound via light is beyond the scope of this chapter. At its basic level, however, the sound wave modulates the IR signal by pulsing the LED on and off in the transmitter. In effect, the pulsing pattern is "carried" on the invisible, modulated IR signal. The receiver contains a fish-eye lens and receiver diode that is sensitive to IR light from multiple directions. The receiver demodulates (or extracts) the sound wave from the modulated IR signal. Once the sound wave has been extracted, it can be delivered to headphones, or some other ear coupling method. IR technology works very well indoors in well-lit and darkened rooms, but direct sunlight can interfere with transmission. Just as an object can block our vision, IR is similarly affected by objects and there must be no obstruction between the transmitter LED and receiver diode.

The stethoset receiver (Figure 8–1) and headphones (Figure 8–2) have all of the needed electronics built in and can receive an IR signal directly. The pocket-sized receiver (Figure 8–3) is similar to an FM receiver. These types of receivers can be used with earphones, hearing aids, or cochlear implants. Without hearing aids or cochlear implants, a mono or stereo set of earphones can be plugged directly into the receiver. If used with hearing aids or cochlear implants, the IR signal can be sent via neckloop to the telecoil inside the amplification device. Finally, a cochlear implant can also be hard wired to the pocket-sized receiver with a direct audio input (DAI) patch cord. This combination of connections between the receiver and amplification device, or receiver direct to the ears, will be manufacturer and model dependent. One will need to be sure to check the connection possibilities on the particular devices in question.

With the development of frequency-modulation (FM), Wi-Fi, LAN, Bluetooth, LTE, and other wireless transmission technologies, the use of IR for assisted listening has declined in recent years. Some will say that the need for a separate receiver which then couples with amplification devices is a disadvantage of IR technology. An intermediary device is needed, however, because there is no hearing aid or implantable device with a built-in IR receiver. Next, the receiver must be in direct line of sight of the transmitter, limiting the locations in which IR will work well. In different areas within a room, for example, without direct line

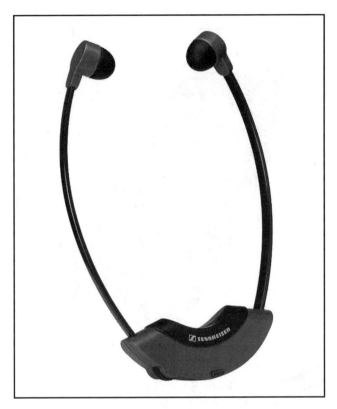

Figure 8–1. Sennheiser RI 150. Image courtesy of Sennheiser.

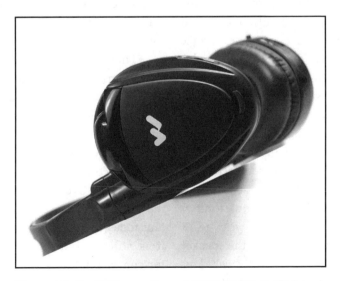

Figure 8–2. Williams Sound WIR RX15-2 IR head-phone receiver. Image courtesy of Williams Sound.

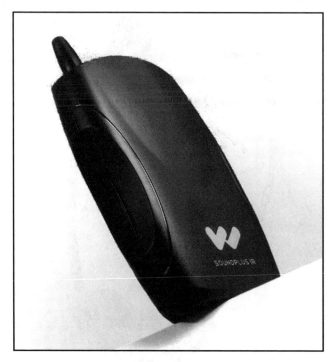

Figure 8–3. Williams Sound WIR RX22-4 IR receiver. Image courtesy of Williams Sound.

of sight there could be some loss of the transmitted signal. Finally, recall that direct sunlight can cause interference with IR transmissions. Other technologies not affected by sunlight (e.g., FM and induction) would be advised over IR in those applications. Having stated these limitations, there is anecdotal evidence that at least the direct-line-of-sight disadvantage may not be strictly true. For example, Steve Boone (personal communication, 2014) cited situations at conferences that individuals wearing IR receivers with their backs to the speaker could hear the speech perfectly well. This situation occurred because the IR waves,

much like sound waves, reflected off the walls in that room and were picked up by the receiver.

There are a number of advantages to IR systems as assistive technology. First, two IR systems can be used in adjacent rooms simultaneously without interference from each other because the signal (i.e., light) cannot travel through walls. Although the development of multiple channel assistive listening devices may make that lack of interference less important today than it was in earlier decades, it is still an important consideration for commercial uses. Second, IR can be used in rooms of almost any size because additional transmitters can be connected together for coverage of larger spaces. Third, because sound is being sent from transmitters to receivers at the speed of light, there is no delay in reception of the signal. This is important in several venues, including live theaters, movie theaters, and in-home television viewing so that the sound is synchronized with the image or actors. Fourth, the signal integrity is preserved very well in IR technology, meaning the listener will receive a clean signal, a fact quite important for users with hearing loss.

Assistive Listening Applications

Personal Use

Several companies produce IR devices suitable for home use including television viewing and radio and stereo listening. In general these instruments are composed of a transmitter, or base stand, and stethoset headphones. The transmitter functions as the charging unit for the battery that powers the receiver. The transmitter has an electrical cord as well as a cord that plugs into the television, radio, or stereo system. The headset requires a battery and most, if not all, units now have a rechargeable battery, which recharges automatically when the headset is placed in the base unit. Some companies may have a second, spare rechargeable battery housed within the transmitter. The exact type of rechargeable battery may vary

by company and product, for example a lithium-ion or lithium-polymer battery. A single, full charge, which can take from 3 to 14 hours, may provide anywhere from 6 to 16 hours of use, again depending on the manufacturer, model, and battery. Some companies offer automatic on/off; that is, when the stethoset headphones are removed from the base the device automatically turns on; returning the headphones to the base shuts off the unit. Other companies have a single on-off-volume control located on the stethoset receiver.

The outgoing audio signal from the television, satellite, cable box, radio, or stereo is converted to light and sent out of the transmitter to the IR receiver. In home transmission applications, this light beam from transmitter to receiver is sent on one of two carrier frequencies, either 2.3 or 2.8 MHz. The actual receiver on the stethoset headphones is located on the cross-piece that hangs beneath the listener's chin. Controls that may be found on IR receivers include volume control and balance control. The volume control is used to raise and lower the overall sound level of the IR receiver. Often, the television volume control remains separate so that individuals other than the person wearing the receiver can adjust the TV volume to a comfortable level, then the person with the IR device can adjust his or her individual sound level. The balance control will change the volume of the sound between the right and left ears. Figure 8–4 contains a drawing of the typical in-home setup for an IR television viewing application.

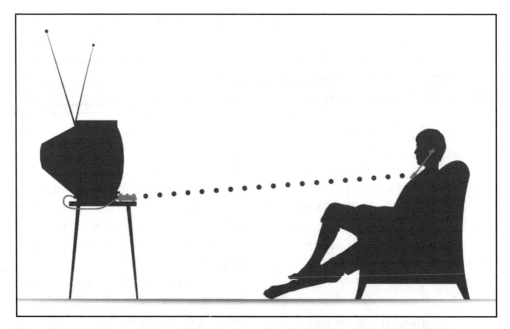

Figure 8–4. In-home infrared application setup. Image courtesy of TV Ears.

Personal Use Infrared Product Samples

In this section we present a few examples of in-home IR devices from different companies. Inclusion is not necessarily an endorsement of these products or companies.

Sennheiser

The Sennheiser Set 830-TV (Figure 8–5) is designed to work specifically with television sets. The receiver weighs 2.4 ounces (68 grams), has a large volume control wheel in front, a maximum sound pressure level (SPL) of 125 dB SPL (~105 dB HL), and up to 12 hours' operating time on a full, 3-hour charge. To turn the receiver

"on" the earpieces are pulled apart; the receiver has an automatic shutoff function 30 seconds after removal from the ears. Sennheiser includes warnings about high sound volume and cautions the user to turn the volume down before inserting the earpieces and not to expose himself or herself to continuous high volume levels. The transmitter, or base, operates at either 2.3 or 2.8 MHz with a range of up to 39 feet (12 meters) and has an on-off switch that lights up green when it is turned on. This unit can broadcast in stereo or mono and has intensity compression and treble adjustments. The compression appears to be wide dynamic range compression (WDRC), while the treble adjustment will boost the higher frequencies between about 10 and 20 dB, as shown in Figure 8–6.

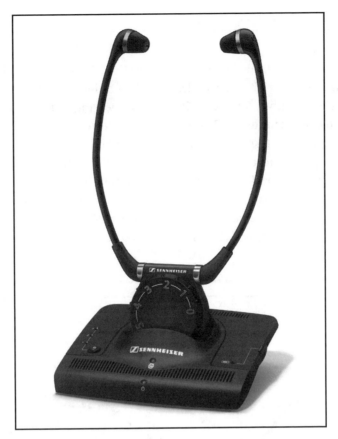

Figure 8–5. Sennheiser Set 830-TV. Image courtesy of Sennheiser.

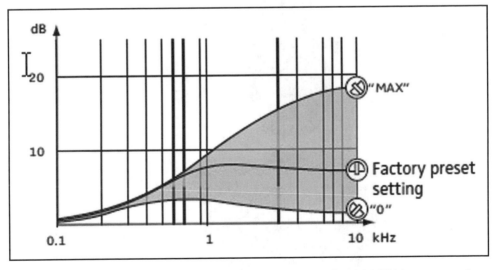

Figure 8–6. Sennheiser treble boost spectrum for the Set 830-TV. Image courtesy of Sennheiser.

The Sennheiser Set 830-S (Figure 8–7) also works at either 2.3 or 2.8 MHz. The receiver weighs only 1.8 ounces (50 grams) and can operate for up to 12 hours when fully charged. The transmitter base has a range of up to 39 feet (12 meters). This particular product package includes a lithium-polymer rechargeable battery, a lanyard to hold the receiver around the neck, and the Sennheiser EZT 3011 induction loop. The induction loop sends the signal from the 830-S receiver to any hearing aid with a telecoil. The 830-S receiver will also connect directly to headphones. The listener can take the 830-S receiver to any public setting in which IR technology is used and which is operated on either the 2.3 MHz channel or the 2.8 MHz channel. The Sennheiser Set 900 is like the Set 830-S in almost all

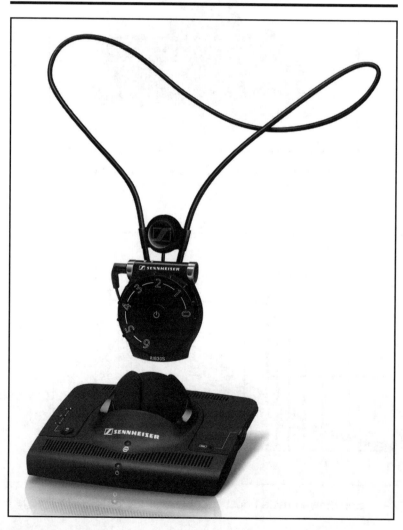

Figure 8–7. Sennheiser Set 830-S. Image courtesy of Sennheiser.

particulars but with the addition of two switchable microphones on the receiver. These microphones allow the wearer to amplify the voice of a communication partner or to improve the listener's awareness of their surroundings, for example, to hear the telephone ring or the doorbell sound, while using the receiver.

TV Ears

The TV Ears company specializes in devices for in-home use. TV Ears markets analog and digital devices (Figures 8–8 and 8–9, respectively). The analog systems are designed for use with televisions that have analog audio out ports; however, these devices may also be used with cable and satellite boxes. The transmitter functions as the charger for the stethoset receiver. Users are told to charge the receiver for at least 14 hours before the first use of the system. On a full charge the receiver will provide about 6 hours of listening but will vary depending on the volume setting. The TV Ears headset receiver has a single "on-off-volume" dial as well as a tone control. The tone control

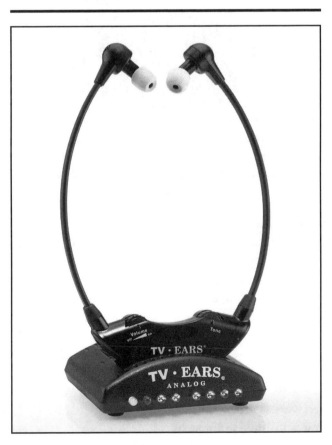

Figure 8–8. TV Ears Analog System. Image courtesy of TV Ears.

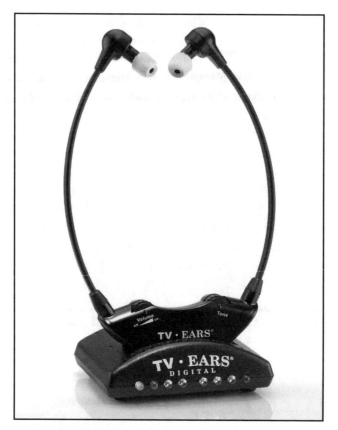

Figure 8–9. TV Ears Digital System. Image courtesy of TV Ears.

will vary the bass and treble frequency regions reaching the listener's ears. The TV Ears 5.0 digital systems are quite similar to the analog version with the exception that these are used with televisions that have digital audio out ports.

Williams Sound

Williams Sound sells IR transmitters (and emitters) and receivers as separate units, allowing consumers to "mix and match" to achieve the best system for their particular application. Also available are two-channel (WIR TX925 SoundPlus) and four-channel (WIR TX900 SoundPlus) turnkey systems, which can be used as portable units or permanently installed. Williams Sound has three types of receivers (not sold with a dedicated transmitter) that can be used in home applications and taken to public venues: the Sound-Plus headphones (WIR RX15-2; see Figure 8–2), the WIR RX22-4N 4-channel receiver (see Figure 8–3), and the Sound-Plus stethoset-style earphones (WIR RX18; Figure 8–10). The two-channel receivers will operate on 2.3 or 2.8 MHz

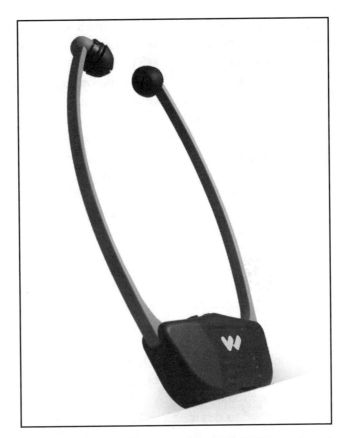

Figure 8–10. Williams Sound WIR RX18 stethoset receiver. Image courtesy of Williams Sound.

and the four-channel adds 3.3 and 3.8 MHz. The stethoset will also operate in stereo mode.

Wide Area Applications

Wide area applications can be implemented in many different spaces including courtrooms, houses of worship, concert halls, live theaters, movie theaters, museums, conference centers, and many others. The basic setup in wide area applications is similar to that for in-home applications. A transmitter, often referred to as an emitter in these applications, or several emitters, are plugged into the sound source, most likely the existing sound system. The signal is carried within the transmitted light beam to the IR receivers worn by individual audience members. Some companies that offer this type of equipment are AuDex, Sennheiser, and Williams Sound. The U.S. Department of Justice has specific standards for wide area applications regarding the seating capacity of the area, the minimum number of required receivers, and how many of those receivers must be hearing aid compatible. In areas with 50 or fewer seats there must be at least two receivers, both of which must be hearing aid compatible. As the number of seats increases, the number of receivers increases, and in venues with more than 200 seats, 25% of the receivers must be hearing aid compatible, as can be seen in Table 8–1.

Perhaps the most important piece of advice we can give regarding these systems is to contact these companies or their product representatives for professional help in installing wide area IR systems. These companies do have some turnkey systems, that is, systems designed for use in a particular kind of space, a courtroom, for example (Figure 8–11). In this case one can simply purchase that system, remove it from the box, install, and use. The more likely scenario, however, is that a system will need to be created specifically for the space to fit the needs for that venue and use. We present one example of a turnkey system and one custom system.

Williams Sound offers the SoundPlus Deluxe Courtroom System (WIR SYS3; see Figure 8 11), which is a two-channel IR listening system. Included in this package are an emitter that provides 10,000 square feet of coverage in single-channel mode, three under-the-chin receivers, one body receiver, a receiver charger that holds up to five receiver headsets, one induction neckloop, a rack-mountable modulator, a rack mount kit, a wall/ceiling mount, and an Americans with Disabilities Act (ADA) wall plaque. The plaque is included for display to inform patrons that the system in use adheres to ADA requirements. A second emitter can be attached to the primary emitter to enlarge the coverage area.

Sennheiser offers turnkey systems for specific applications as well; however, a buyer can mix and match pieces that will fit that their precise need, too. For example, the SI 30 transmitter (Figure 8–12) will cover up to 750 square feet and operates on 2.3 or 2.8 MHz. Up to three "slave emitters" can be used in conjunction with the SI 30 to increase the coverage area

Table 8–1. Receivers for Assistive Listening Systems

Seating Capacity of Assembly Area	Minimum Number of Required Receivers	Minimum Number of Receivers Required to Be Hearing Aid Compatible
50 or less	2	2
51 to 200	2, plus 1 per 25 seats over 50 seats	2
201 to 500	2, plus 1 per 25 seats over 50 seats	1 per 4 receivers
501 to 1,000	20, plus 1 per 33 seats over 500 seats	1 per 4 receivers
1,001 to 2,000	35, plus 1 per 50 seats over 1000 seats	1 per 4 receivers
2,001 and over	55 plus 1 per 100 seats over 2000 seats	1 per 4 receivers

Source: Adapted from Table 219.3 Receivers for Assistive Listening Systems (US DOJ, 2010).

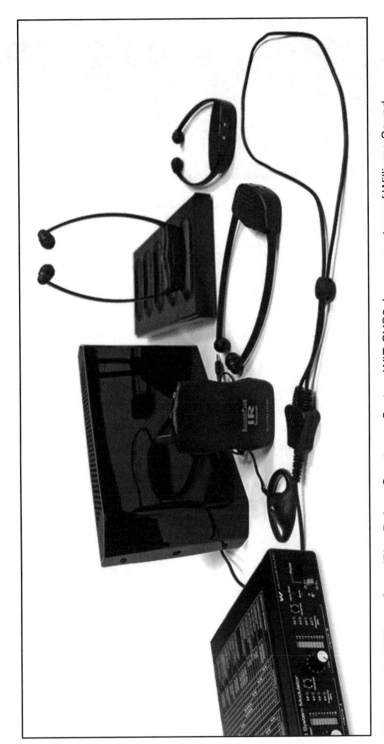

Figure 8–11. Williams SoundPlus Deluxe Courtroom System WIR SYS3. Image courtesy of Williams Sound.

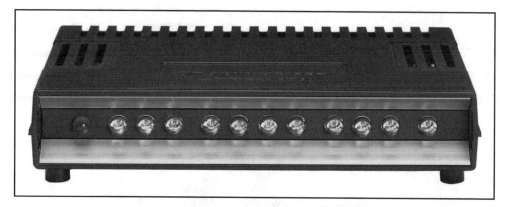

Figure 8–12. Sennheiser SI 30. Image courtesy of Sennheiser.

up to 3,000 square feet. Sennheiser recommends this particular device for use in houses of worship, conference rooms, and courtrooms. Several different receivers can be used with the SI 30, including the stethoset-style, two-channel HDI 830 and the stethoset, single-channel RI 150 (see Figure 8–1). The expertise needed in this situation would include where to place the additional emitters to maximize the coverage area and which receiver or receivers would be best for the venue and use under consideration.

IR has declined in the last several years, IR remains a viable technology for many venues and in many applications. There are a number of IR products available for assisted listening, some designed for personal and in-home use as well as systems designed for wide area and public spaces.

Reference

U.S. Department of Justice. (2010). Table 219.3 Receivers for Assistive Listening Systems. Department of Justice. Retrieved from http://www.ada.gov/regs2010/2010ADAStandards/2010ADAStandards.pdf

Summary

There are advantages and disadvantages to using IR systems. Although the use of

9

Contemporary Wireless Hearing Technologies

Introduction

This chapter differs from most others in this book because much of the application of the technology presented in this chapter is in its infancy. As wireless assistive and access technologies involving frequency modulation (FM), induction hearing loop systems, and infrared (IR) systems are well established (see Chapters 6 through 8) with the potential to grow, the information in this chapter reflects the rapidly progressing wireless technologies used in mobile phones, cordless phones, smart cards, Wi-Fi, and hearing aids, to name a few. Current wireless communication technology capabilities

can both amaze and intimidate users. With almost every electronic device on the market developing or using wireless radio communications (e.g., Bluetooth enabled), it is difficult to keep up with all of the possibilities to improve listening via these communications. This chapter is an introduction to and brief explanation of the industrial, scientific, and medical (ISM) frequency band, Digital Enhanced Cordless Telecommunications (DECT) technology, Global System for Mobile (GSM) Communications technology, near field communication (NFC) technology, and innovations and applications of these wireless communication technologies. While it may not be as critical for us to have the same degree of understanding of these technologies as someone in the information technology (IT) field, it is important to understand some of the strengths and weaknesses of these methods of wireless communications to understand their possible usefulness as assistive technologies for our clients.

Industrial, Scientific, and Medical (ISM) Radio Band

As the name implies, the industrial, scientific, and medical (ISM) radio band is a band of frequencies (i.e., frequency range) designated for the transmission of radio communications for devices used in the industrial sector, scientific community, and the medical field. These devices can range from microwave ovens to cordless phones, from blood pressure monitors to methods of welding plastic material, and from military radar to industrial heaters. You may have noticed the signs in medical facilities prohibiting mobile phone use. This is because equipment communicating over ISM bands may interrupt other signals that are also being transmitted over the same frequency. Interruption of a signal is referred to as electromagnetic interference. Additionally, some wireless fidelity (e.g., Wi-Fi) networks transmit via the ISM band. These networks are a potential source of electromagnetic interference for mobile devices and vice versa. However, the uses appear limitless for this worldwide accepted frequency band designation. Even progress in future space exploration may rely on using the ISM radio band.

Bluetooth

So what is Bluetooth? Why is it so popular? And, how did it get its name? With its name and functionality tied to a king and a Hollywood starlet, respectively, Bluetooth, whose logo is presented in Figure 9–1, is a form of wireless communication in the ISM band. Specifically, Bluetooth is a secure, short-range (approximately 30 feet), wireless communication between Bluetooth-enabled devices such as televisions, mobile phones, computers, smart devices, and so forth. Bluetooth allows for these devices to be connected without the need for cumbersome, tangle-prone, connector-port specific cables. Its popularity rests in its availability, low power consumption, and low cost. Bluetooth-enabled devices work the same anywhere in the world; they require very little, if any, additional power. Bluetooth-enabled devices are likely to cost more than non-Bluetooth devices, but once this technology becomes common within a type of device, the Bluetooth-enabled devices are not likely to be any more expensive because of Bluetooth (Bluetooth Basics, n.d.). Bluetooth gets its name from a 10th century Danish king, King Harald Blåtand "Bluetooth" Gormsson. He brought together the divided and warring groups from different parts of Scandinavia. Like King Blåtand, illustrated in Figure 9–2, who united people around Scandinavia, Bluetooth technology unites devices via wireless short-range communications (Bluetooth Fast-Facts, n.d.).

Bluetooth can be thought of as the technology of the new millennium. Just

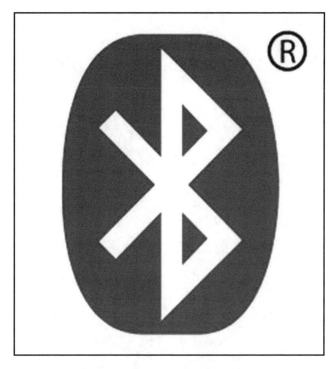

Figure 9–1. The Bluetooth logo. Image courtesy of Bluetooth Special Interest Group.

before the turn of the century, in 1998, a few companies established the Bluetooth Special Interest Group (SIG). By 2001, Bluetooth technology had been developed for mobile phones, personal computers, and hands-free car kits. The technology made it to televisions in 2007 and has progressed at a rapid pace since. A new version of Bluetooth, known as Bluetooth Smart, was introduced in 2011 (History of Bluetooth, n.d.) and provides wireless communication with less energy consumption by Bluetooth-enabled devices.

Many modern hearing aids are Bluetooth or Bluetooth Smart enabled. While there are other types of wireless connec-

tions between devices and hearing aids, the Bluetooth designation identifies the specific uniform structure for devices to connect and communicate with each other. Spaced 1 MHz apart, Bluetooth signals are transmitted over 79 channels on the 2.4 GHz ISM radio band; Bluetooth Low Energy LE uses 40 channels spaced 2 MHz apart. When two devices identify and establish communications with each other via Bluetooth, a process referred to as "discovery and handshake," the two devices are then "paired" and can communicate (e.g., exchange files like word documents, photos, and songs). When one or more devices are connected to one

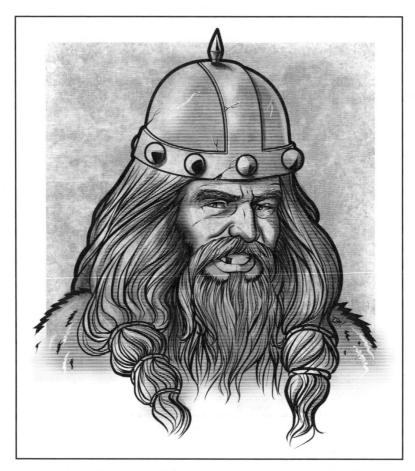

Figure 9–2. An artist's rendering of King Blantand (Bluetooth). Illustration courtesy of Timothy Lim, AuD.

another, they make up a *piconet*. A piconet can be thought of as the network connecting these devices at any moment in time. When one device is brought into or removed from the functional range of the other devices, it is either added to or removed from the piconet. A maximum of eight devices can be added to a piconet. One device, the master of a piconet, can communicate with up to seven other devices, or slaves. An interesting feature is that any device, master or slave, can belong to multiple piconets at the same time. A collection of piconets is referred to as a *scatternet*. This ability of networks to grow allows almost limitless connectivity options (Bluetooth Basics, n.d.). When at least one of the devices in a piconet, like a computer or smart device, can connect to the Internet, the network connecting the devices is referred to as an *Internet of Things* (IoT). An illustration of an IoT is provided in Figure 9–3. An example of an application of an IoT includes the

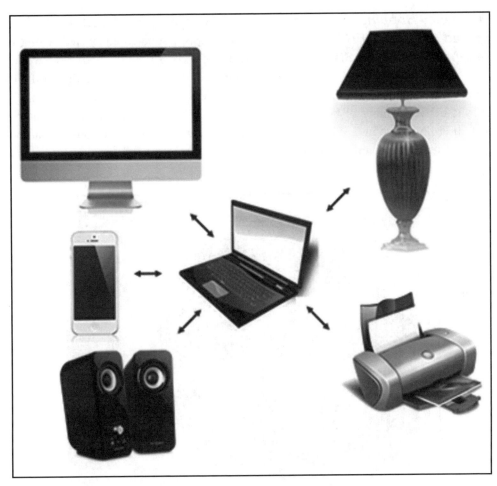

Figure 9–3. Wireless devices connected in a piconet, or small network. Because the piconet has access to connect to the Internet, it is also referred to as an Internet of Things (IoT).

ability to use a Bluetooth device to control another device via the Internet, like turning the lights on or off in your home while you are away.

Global System for Mobile Technology

Global System for Mobile (GSM) technology is probably familiar to anyone with a mobile phone. This technology allows devices, such as mobile phones, to communicate via networks. These networks can vary in size, from large networks, known as *macro cells*, to small networks, known as femto cells. Macro cells require the large antennas which have become common on tall buildings or hilltops. Femto cells are considerably smaller and are typically designed for residential use.

Frequency Hopping Spread Spectrum (FHSS) Technology and the Starlet

The security of the wireless communications between many of these devices, including Bluetooth and Wi-Fi, are safeguarded using an adaptive form of frequency hopping spread spectrum (FHSS), which was first patented by Hedy Lamarr (Figure 9–4), a 1930 to 1950s Hollywood starlet, and her neighbor, George Antheil, a music composer (Brilliant, Beautiful, & Bold, n.d.) in 1942. These two inventors used a player piano (also called an autopiano) as the model for this ingenious

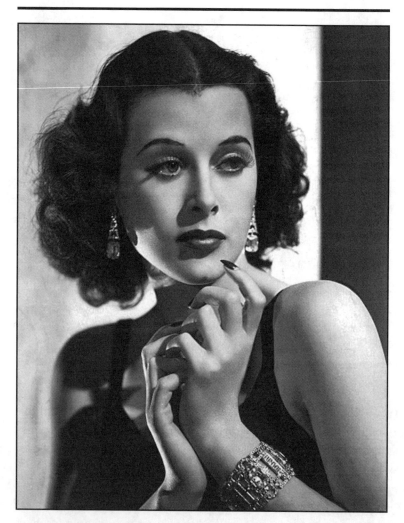

Figure 9–4. Actress/inventor Hedy Lamarr is credited with patenting Frequency Hopping Spread Spectrum (FHSS) technology. Image courtesy of Wikimedia Commons.

idea, but it had nothing to do with Wi-Fi or mobile phones, since neither had been invented at the time. A player piano used perforated music sheets or metallic rolls to strike the notes and produce the music automatically.

The way FHSS works is that one device pseudo-randomly hops from one carrier frequency to another once synchronized (or synched) with another device. The devices are synchronized, much like the relationship between the player piano and its instruction sheet (i.e., sheet music). The piano plays the keys it is told to play by the instruction sheet, with only the piano and the instruction sheet knowing the sequence and timing of the notes to be played. The first intended application for the frequency hopping patent was for naval warfare. At the time, naval vessels had difficulty navigating fired torpedoes via radio waves without radio interference from the enemy. Lamarr and Antheil proposed sending the navigation signals over multiple carrier frequencies, but the signals would hop from one carrier frequency to another in a manner that only the sender and receiver (torpedo) knew and to which they were both synchronized. The relationship between the torpedo and the transmitter was similar to that of the piano and instruction sheet. This technology later evolved into FHSS (Brilliant, Beautiful, & Bold, n.d.).

Streaming Devices

There are some Bluetooth devices designed to receive a signal but with no intent or capacity to return a signal. When this one-way transmission occurs, it is referred to as *streaming*. A commercially available hearing aid accessory/streaming device is illustrated in Figure 9–5.

Streaming requires the second device to receive a signal, but it does not require that device be able to transmit a signal. We stream when listening to music from our smartphone or smart device via Bluetooth-enabled headphones or speakers. We stream the audio directions from our GPS systems to our Bluetooth-enabled audio systems in cars. In both of these examples, there is no return signal, only the one-way signal allowing us to listen to music or driving directions. With hearing aids the streaming device is often placed in a pocket or worn around the neck. The streaming device transmits to the hearing aids from another device, such as a mobile phone (Figure 9–6A). Because of the reduced energy consumption of Bluetooth LE, hearing aids have the capacity to interact with external devices without a streaming device (Figure 9–6B). While potentially intimidating to many hearing aid wearers, this technology is quite user friendly. For example, when the hearing aids have been "paired" with another device, they will recognize one another each time they are in close enough proximity. When "paired" with a mobile phone, the hearing aid wearer can hear the phone ring directly through their hearing aids. To answer the phone, the hearing aid wearer simply presses the designated button on the streaming device (Burrows, 2010).

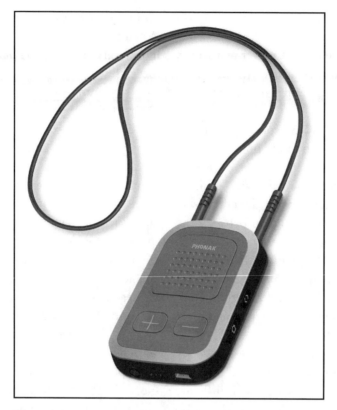

Figure 9–5. The Phonak ComPilot works as a streaming device as it transmits its signal to hearing aids over the ISM band. Image courtesy of Phonak.

Near Field Communications

Transmitting via the 13.56 MHz band, near field communication (NFC) is another method of wireless communication. Similar to Bluetooth, NFC is a short-range communication technology but is newer and less well-known. Like Bluetooth, NFC technology has been incorporated into smart devices, except there are a few differences between the two technologies. While Bluetooth requires a few seconds and power for secure pairing,

NFC operates using a *point-to-point system*. Point-to-point connections, between two devices with NFC tags, allow communications between the sender and receiver to be established without the need for pairing. Thus, establishing a line of communication for NFC devices is almost instantaneous. In addition, NFC devices require less power than Bluetooth devices for these connections. Essentially, all that is required for two NFC devices to communicate is for one device to enter the proximity of the other. Additionally,

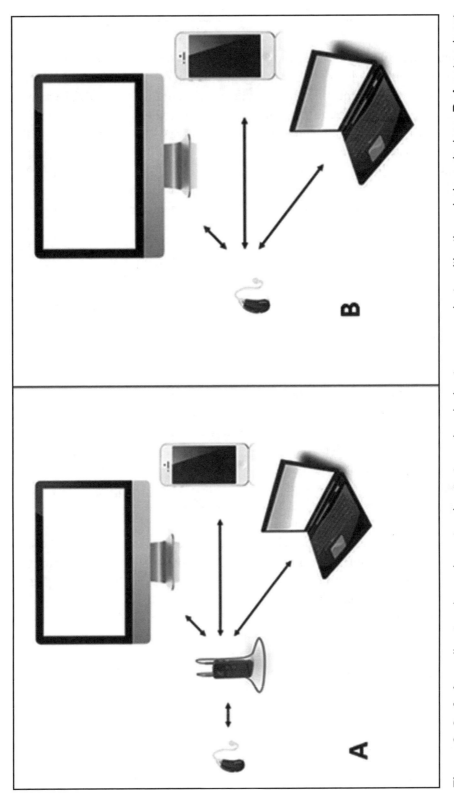

Figure 9–6. A. A small network, or piconet, using a streaming device to communicate with other wireless devices. **B.** A network not requiring a streaming device to communicate with other wireless devices. These piconets can be considered an Internet of Things (IoT), as they are connected to the Internet via the laptop computer or smartphone.

NFC devices have a much shorter range of transmission and are better suited for transmitting small amounts of information. Examples of NFC use, other than in hearing assistive devices, include the transfer of images or video from one device to another, like bumping phones with a friend to share games or video. Electronic mobile NFC allows for such things as the payment for goods or services via noncontact credit cards or electronic tickets, like swiping your smartphone at a checkout line. Another example includes the use of wallet- or keychain-size smart cards at a gas pump, by simply waving the card in front of the sensor, to pay for your gas. Presently, NFC technology is applied in some hearing aids to allow the left and right hearing aids to communicate with one another. This technology supports "superdirectional" microphone technology discussed in Chapter 4. NFC technology is also being used in various assistive listening devices. Locations suited for assistive listening devices using NFC-based technology include museums and art galleries, as information can be delivered near exhibits without carrying over and causing interference at other exhibits in the vicinity (About Near Field Communication, n.d.).

Digital Enhanced Cordless Telecommunications

The microwave technology known as Digital Enhanced Cordless Telecommunications (DECT) uses yet another frequency designated for wireless communications. DECT uses the 1.9 GHz band and is less susceptible to interference than technology operating on the ISM band. Presently, the most common use of DECT technology appears to be in cordless phones and baby monitors. Using a base station, the signal is routed to each device within a distance of about 600 meters (~1,950 feet), large enough to cover a sizable building. As was mentioned in Chapter 4, a hearing aid wearer may be able to listen bilaterally with a DECT phone (Figure 9–7) rather than through just one hearing aid at a time. While present application is limited to certain hearing aid manufacturers, DECT technology is improving. In a similar manner as Bluetooth, improved energy consumption in Bluetooth-enabled devices with Bluetooth Smart, a low energy consuming version of DECT, known as DECT ultra low energy (ULE), is now available.

Summary

This chapter covered some of the different ways in which devices communicate wirelessly over different frequency bands. The ISM band covers 2.4 GHz, while DECT and NFC operate over 1.9 GHz and 13.56 MHz, respectively. These differences result in advantages (e.g., increased range), disadvantages (e.g., potential interference), and limitations (e.g., government licensing) for each of these bands of communications and types of technology. Within the ISM band, Bluetooth technology and handshake pairing use frequency hopping for minimal interference and streaming between

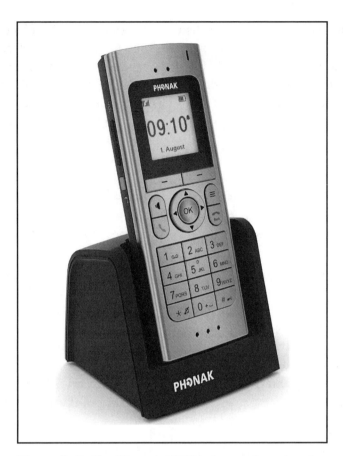

Figure 9–7. The Phonak DECT phone allows hearing aid wearers to hear phone conversations through both hearing aids. Image courtesy of Phonak.

different devices or between devices and the Internet. A network of devices, called a piconet, can be connected to the Internet to create an Internet of things, or IoT. Bluetooth technology can deliver audio from mobile phones, MP3 players, and televisions to a hearing aid wearer with minimal interference.

While Bluetooth uses pairing and frequency hopping, NFC uses point-to-point communications and NFC tags. By having pre-established identification between devices via NFC tags, initial connection between devices is quicker than Bluetooth. An additional feature of NFC is less energy consumption, compared to Bluetooth. The effective range for NFC is smaller than that of Bluetooth and DECT, but allows for applications, like smart cards or communication between bilateral hearing aids. DECT devices operate around a base unit which allows communication between devices within range, similar to Wi-Fi technology. The range can vary but typically is larger than the range of Bluetooth. Some specially designed DECT phones allow hearing aid wearers to hear phone conversations through both hearing aids.

References

About Near Field Communication. (n.d.). Retrieved from http://www.nearfield communication.org/about-nfc.html

Bluetooth basics: A look at the basics of Bluetooth Technology. (n.d.). Retrieved from http://www.bluetooth .com/Pages/Basics.aspx

Brilliant, Beautiful, & Bold: Hedy Lamarr, the official site. (n.d.). Retrieved from http://www.hedylamarr.com/about/ biography.html

Burrows, D. L. (2010). Bluetooth technology in hearing aids: A clinician's perspective. *Perspectives on Audiology, 6,* 4–8. doi:10.1044/poa6.1.4

DECT—Worldwide technology for voice and data application. (n.d.). Retrieved from http://www.dect.org/dect-tech nology

Fast facts: Welcome to Bluetooth Technology 101, A brief tutorial on Bluetooth wireless technology. (n.d.). Retrieved from http://www.bluetooth .com/Pages/Fast-Facts.aspx

NFC for Beginners Part 4—Difference between NFC and Bluetooth. (n.d.). Retrieved from http://receivetipstricks. hubpages.com/hub/nfc-vs-bluetooth

Our history: History of the Bluetooth Special Interest Group. (n.d.). Retrieved from http://www.bluetooth.com/Pages /History-of-Bluetooth.aspx

PART III

Telecommunications and Related Technologies

10

Telecommunications Access[1]

Overview

The Communications Act of 1934 established what we now know as the Federal Communications Commission (FCC), which regulates a variety of interstate and international communications. Although this act has been around for a while, it took several more acts of the U.S. Congress over the last 80 years to achieve the level of accessibility for telephones, mobile phones, and related telecommunication services that we see today. In particular, the Twenty-First Century Communications and Video Accessibility Act (CVAA) of 2010 brought previous accessibility laws of the 1980s and 1990s up to date with more current technologies. More information about the CVAA can be found in Chapter 2.

In this chapter, we focus primarily on speech-based telecommunication technologies for individuals with hearing loss who are able to use their own voice and their own ears. It is expected that some of these individuals have milder forms of hearing loss and do not wear hearing aids, while others have more severe hearing losses and will be using a hearing aid or implantable device to use a telephone or mobile phone. For individuals with milder forms of hearing loss, a phone with built-in volume and tone controls

---

[1] Portions of this chapter are reprinted or modified from a previously published article by Atcherson, S. R., & Highley, P. (2013, Spring). Cell phones decoded. *Hearing Health*, *29*(2), 22–27. Permission of Hearing Health Foundation.

may be all that is needed, but several other options are also available for those who need it. We would be remiss, however, if we did not also provide some information about visual-based telecommunication technologies for individuals with hearing loss who cannot speak well, are uncomfortable using their voice, or elect not to use their voice. There are visual text- and sign language-based telecommunication services that may be appropriate for and/or preferred by these individuals.

Speech-Based Telecommunications

For conventional acoustic telephone communications, the Hearing Aid Compatibility (HAC) Act of 1988 gave the FCC authority to require that all "essential" telephones be hearing aid compatible. Essential phones are defined as coin-operated telephones, telephones provided for emergency use, and other telephones frequently needed for use by persons using such hearing aids. Landline (hardwired) phones were well covered by this act; however, mobile and wireless phones were not part of that original regulation. Rather, mobile and wireless phones were exempt for a period of time. In 2003, the FCC determined that the exemption for mobile and wireless phones, which were growing in popularity and becoming more affordable, would severely limit accessibility for individuals with hearing loss. Because of this determination, the FCC began establishing rules for hearing aid compatibility for digital wireless phones. In more recent years, the FCC regulations have been tweaked further with mandates that cellular providers carry a certain number of hearing aid compatible mobile phones and/or some minimum quality/rating of hearing aid compatibility under test standards. In this section, we provide an overview of acoustic and inductive coupling, a discussion of hearing aid compatibility (applicable also for many implantable devices), and some resources and tips for consideration.

Acoustic and Inductive Coupling

There are two principal methods by which desired signals can be picked up by the miniature electronics of a hearing aid or implantable device (see also Chapter 7). The first method, *acoustic coupling*, is through a tiny microphone that picks up airborne sounds in the environment. In this case, the airborne sound is coming from the telephone speaker and is routed into the hearing aid microphone. Acoustic coupling may work fine for some individuals unless there is a lot of background noise in the environment, such as a busy street or other people talking. To achieve optimal acoustic coupling, the phone speaker must be held as closely as possible to the microphone of the hearing aid or implantable device. One potential downside of the acoustic coupling method is that some hearing aids may begin to whistle (feedback) whenever a phone is placed next to them.

The second method, *inductive coupling*, is through a different electronic part of the hearing aid or implantable device, called a *telecoil*, which may need to be added. Chapter 7 covers the more technical aspects of telecoils, but here we describe their use more specifically for telephones. A telecoil is built into many hearing aid and implantable device models and is a small coil of wire no more than a few millimeters in length (see Figure 7–1). When turned on, the telecoil acts as an antenna and is sensitive to electromagnetic signals in various audio equipment. The electromagnetic leakage described here is not necessarily a bad thing. For example, if a phone or even a pair of headphones has an audio signal coming out of its speaker, it may also produce sufficient electromagnetic energy that carries the same speech or music signal. When this electromagnetic leakage is picked up by a telecoil, inductive coupling is achieved. The interesting thing about inductive coupling is that only the signal from the phone or other audio device is picked up, without interference from acoustic noise in the environment (again a busy street or other people talking). This is possible if the microphone is purposely deactivated when the telecoil is turned on. Telecoils can also be used with certain personal and public assistive listening devices (ALDs), including hearing loop systems (see Chapters 6 through 8). The reason that some hearing aids may not have a telecoil could be due to space limitations. Alternatively, some hearing aids and implantable devices may have a telecoil, but it would need to be activated and programmed by a hearing professional, such as an audiologist. To ensure that the telecoil offers gain comparable

to the microphone, the telecoil should be programmed and verified (see Chapter 7). In some hearing aids, an autophone or autotelecoil feature may be available. For example, the telecoil may automatically be activated when the electromagnetic leakage of a phone is detected. If a particular phone does not automatically activate the telecoil, small stick-on magnets may be placed on the phone handset to assist.

One pitfall of telecoils is that they may not be immune to other sources of interference in the environment. For example, certain fluorescent room lighting, computer monitors, theft protection systems, and even the backlight of a mobile phone can cause radio frequency (RF) emission buzzing. Sometimes the solution is as easy as moving to a different location. Other times, the problem may be due to a malfunction of the other devices listed or even the hearing aid circuitry. In other words, all forms of electronics can have failures.

Hearing Aid Compatibility

Phone-Specific Microphone and Telecoil Ratings

Whether one chooses the acoustic (microphone) or inductive (telecoil) coupling method to communicate using phones, it will be important to consider just how compatible either of these two methods are with existing phones. Now that we know about the differences in acoustic and inductive coupling methods, we can turn our attention to the discussion of mobile phone RF interference ratings and hearing aid RF immunity ratings, often found on the packaging of mobile phones. Both sources of information are necessary to maximize hearing aid compatibility. Some of this information may be found publicly in an Internet search, and other pieces may require assistance from a phone provider and/or hearing professional. The FCC requires that hearing aid compatible mobile phone providers indicate a quality measure (or rating) of how much RF emission (interference) is produced by the mobile phone.

M-ratings will be important for individuals who plan to use the acoustic coupling method using the microphone of the hearing aids. The ratings will be listed as M1, M2, M3, or M4 with M1 having the greatest interference (least compatible) and M4 having the least interference (most compatible). Aiming for mobile phone M-ratings of M3 or M4 is a good strategy.

T-ratings will be important for individuals who plan to use the inductive coupling method with hearing aids that have a built-in telecoil. Some telecoils need to be programmed or activated by the audiologist, if the telecoil option is available. Similar to M-ratings, the telecoil ratings will be listed as T1, T2, T3, or T4 with T1 having the greatest interference (least compatible) and T4 having the least interference (most compatible). Aiming for mobile phone T-ratings of T3 or T4 is a good strategy. Table 10–1 lists three tips that may be helpful to maximize the use of the telecoil. It should be noted that some mobile phones only have

Table 10–1. Telecoil Tips for Mobile Phone Use

Telecoil Tip	Description
Tip 1	Telecoils are aligned in hearing aids with a particular arrangement (vertical), and it may be in a slightly different location in different hearing aid models. After activating the telecoil in your hearing aid, it may be helpful to take the mobile phone and hover around the hearing aid to find what many refer to as the "sweet spot." It may also help to rotate the mobile phone slightly forward or backward to improve the volume or gain.
Tip 2	If two hearing aids are worn, it may help to activate the telecoil only in the better, or preferred ear, while turning the other hearing aid completely off. This has the effect of cutting out background noise and stray RF emission on one side of the head so that one can focus completely on the conversation. For safety reasons, it may help to keep the other hearing aid for environmental awareness.
Tip 3	Some individuals may benefit from (or prefer) listening to their mobile phone through both hearing aid telecoils at the same time. This is possible with the use of wearable induction earhooks/silhouettes or an induction loop. One may be able to plug this wearable induction accessory directly into the audio jack of the mobile phone. An audiologist or assistive listening device supplier may be able to assist with this option.

M-ratings, whereas others have both M- and T-ratings. As current examples, the ratings for the Samsung Galaxy S5 is M4/T4 (released Spring 2014), while the Apple iPhone 6 is M3/T4 (released Fall 2014). Another great product is the Jitterbug 5 mobile phone designed with senior citizens in mind. It is a flip-style (clamshell) mobile phone with large buttons, a loudspeaker phone, and ideal ratings of M4/T4.

Hearing Aid-Specific Microphone and Telecoil Ratings

If the option is available, one may be able to look up the M- and T-ratings of prospective hearing aid products. Hearing aids less affected by, or immune to, RF emission (interference) in mobile phones would receive a higher rating (i.e., M3, M4, T3, or T4). The American National Standards Institute has a standard (ANSI C63.19) that calls for simple arithmetic to determine the overall quality of hearing aid compatibility by combining the ratings of both phone and hearing aid. For example, a mobile phone with a rating of M3 and a hearing aid rating of M4 produces a combined overall rating of 7 (i.e., M3 + M4 = M7). An overall rating of 4 indicates "usable performance," 5 indicates "normal performance," and 6 or greater indicates "excellent performance." Again, the higher the overall rating, the better the compatibility should be. Unfortunately, M- and T-ratings in hearing aids are not regulated by the FCC and any reporting of these ratings for hearing aids is currently voluntarily offered by the individual hearing aid manufac-

turers. The Food and Drug Administration (FDA) regulates hearing aids and over time we may come to see increased reporting of these ratings.

Considerations for Mobile Phone Purchase

Other than the purchase of hearing aids, perhaps the most important point regarding the purchase of mobile phones is the "try before you buy" strategy. Ask about the store's merchandise return policy if there is a need to take a mobile phone out of the store to try in all other listening situations. If available, experimenting with both acoustic (microphone) and inductive (telecoil) coupling methods is advised. Do not hesitate to ask the mobile phone representative questions about hearing aid compatibility. If there is interest in using the telecoil, it would help to be sure that the telecoil can be activated for use. Additional mobile phone considerations are shown in Table 10–2.

For mobile phone purchases, there are two websites available to prescreen for hearing aid compatibility. One website is http://www.phonescoop.com, and the other is http://www.accesswireless .org. Both of these websites can help you narrow your search for phones by searching for specific features (e.g., hearing aid compatibility, touchscreen) to make the most of your time and effort. To access hearing aid compatibility options with http://www.phonescoop.com, you will need to go to the Phone Finder section of the website, click on the link "show all options" related to Specifications. Under

Table 10–2. Additional Mobile Phone Considerations

Consideration	Description/Explanation
Vibrate mode	This may be helpful when the mobile phone ringer is hard to hear, and it can also double as a wake-up alarm or reminder.
Volume control	Is the mobile phone volume loud enough at its maximum setting? If not, can the hearing aid volume be adjusted or the telecoil strength boosted? See also "Senior mode" below.
Speaker phone	People with mobility or dexterity issues may find that using the mobile phone's speaker may be a better option.
Wireless communication	There may be the option of having mobile phones and hearing aids communicate wirelessly in a hands-free arrangement using Bluetooth streamers, 2.4 GHz (e.g., made for iPhone hearing aids), or comparable wireless technology. Additional devices may be required for this to work.
Video chat	Smartphones with built-in cameras may permit video-based mobile phone calls that allow you to see and hear callers via FaceTime or Skype, two video chat programs. Video chat may work using either cellular service or Wi-Fi.
Senior mode	In some mobile phones a "senior mode" option may be turned on that gives the mobile phone a boost in overall amplification or in the higher pitches.
Text-only phones	Some carriers offer text-only plans that people who find it difficult to hear on mobile phones may prefer to use. These plans do not automatically disable the voice capabilities of the phone for safety reasons, and you may be charged additionally for any voice-related minutes.

Specifications, scroll down and locate Features > Accessibility > Hearing Aid Compatible. To access hearing aid compatibility options with http://www.access wireless.org, click on Phones and access the GARI (Global Accessibility Reporting Initiative) link. Admittedly, neither of these links are user friendly because of the sheer volume of information, but after spending a little time with each website, it will be possible to locate specific phones and their hearing aid compatibility ratings. Although helpful for some, it may be helpful to deselect the other accessibility features (e.g., mobility/dexterity, vision,

and cognitive). If there is a need to restrict a search to certain mobile phone carriers, http://www.phonescoop.com will permit this option. Otherwise, one can check individual mobile phone carriers' websites to read about their individual policies and product listings. (Table 10–3 provides the four major carriers.)

Hardwired Phones

Hardwired phones remain commonplace in the home and office with a landline. Similar to the Jitterbug 5 mobile

Table 10–3. Four Mobile Phone Carrier Websites

Carrier	Website
AT&T	http://www.wireless.att.com/learn/articles-resources/disability-resources/hearing-aid-compatibility.jsp
Sprint	http://www.sprint.com/landings/accessibility/hearing_aid.html
Verizon	http://www.verizonwireless.com/aboutus/accessibility/digitalPhones.html
T-Mobile	https://www.t-mobile.com/Company/CompanyInfo.aspx?tp=Abt_Tab_Consumer Info&tsp=Abt_Sub_AccessibilityPolicy

phone designed with senior citizens in mind, there are a few hardwired amplified phones designed for the same target group, or for any individual with hearing loss. These hardwired phones tend to feature large digital displays, large buttons, a powerful handset for telecoil use, loudspeaker phone, and one or more controls for volume and tone. They may also have a flashing mechanism to alert when the phone is ringing. Figure 10–1 shows one such example of an amplified phone.

Other Methods for Coupling to Phones

The advent of other forms of wireless technology (see Chapter 9) have made it possible for some hearing aid users to move away from telecoil coupling to other forms of coupling. Admittedly, some telecoil users have complained about the buzzing RF sound as well as having to find the "sweet spot," but many have learned to overcome these issues with experience and practice. We also know from Chapter 7 that the low-frequency speech sounds for

the telecoil will be attenuated relative to what one will receive with microphones. What is now available in many newer hearing aids is the ability to use hearing aids as a wireless receiver, not only with mobile phones, but also with a variety of other audio devices (e.g., MP3 player, computers, and tablet devices). Here is an example: Rather than having to hold a mobile phone up to the hearing aid with a telecoil, one may now be able to synchronize a mobile phone to hearing aids and wirelessly transmit the audio directly to the hearing aids in a hands-free fashion. This wireless technology is already available in many hearing aids (e.g., ReSoundLiNX and Starkey Halo, made-for-iPhone hearing aids) using a 2.4 GHz wireless technology, and soon will be available in implantable devices as well. Since the mobile phone may also be the user's portable music and entertainment device, those sounds can also be wirelessly transmitted directly to the hearing aids. Another way to transmit audio to hearing aids is via a neck-worn streamer device (e.g., Oticon ConnectLine and Phonak ComPilot) that synchronizes with various

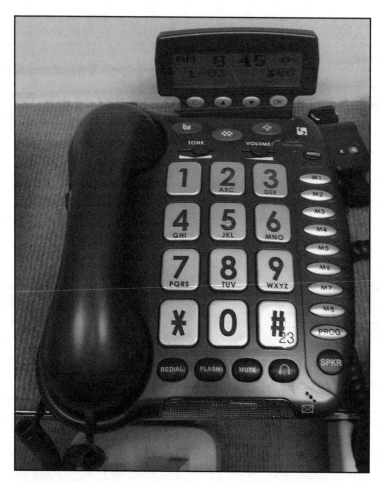

Figure 10–1. Example hardwired amplified phone (ClearSounds CS40XLC). Photo credit: Samuel R. Atcherson, PhD.

Bluetooth-enabled devices. In this case, the specific manner by which the streamer transmits audio to the hearing aids will be manufacturer specific. The possibilities really are endless for a more hands-free approach to audio listening. To learn more about these technologies, interested users should consult with their audiologist. In many ways, the Bluetooth streaming and 2.4 GHz wireless technologies are like frequency-modulated (FM) and induction (via telecoil) wireless technologies, but each with different purposes. FM, particularly dynamic FM, continues to be effective in learning environments, and hearing aid and implant users who have built-in telecoils should always benefit from publicly available induction hearing loop systems without having to carry any additional devices.

Visual-Based Telecommunications

In this chapter, we view visual-based telecommunications as those technologies that involve text or video information, and may or may not also provide audio information. The first technology that comes to mind is the teletypewriter (TTY; Figure 10–2), which is a text-based telephone also sometimes called a Telecommunication Device for the Deaf (TDD). Several individuals are credited for bringing the TTY to its current state including Robert Weitbrecht (Deaf engineer), James C. Marsters (Deaf orthodontist and airline pilot), Paul Taylor (Deaf engineer), and Andrew Saks (Deaf mechanical engineer and grandson of Saks Fifth Avenue founder). Weitbrecht and Marsters developed the PHONETYPE acoustic coupler (modem) and successfully sent the first transmission via long distance back in 1964. Taylor is said to have combined retired Western Union teletypewriters and the acoustic couplers in the late 1960s to create the first TTY and is considered the Father of the Relay Service.

A TTY can permit two callers, each with his or her own TTY device to communicate directly with one another as if

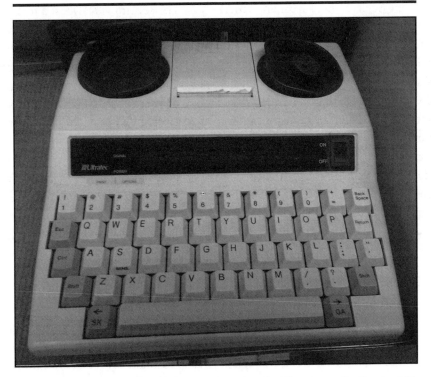

Figure 10–2. Example Teletypewriter (TTY). Photo credit: Samuel R. Atcherson, PhD.

text messaging or instant messaging. The TTY works by encoding letter keystrokes from an electrical signal to a modulated acoustic signal that can be transmitted across telephone lines to be received by another TTY device. The receiving TTY then demodulates the incoming acoustic signal and displays the text electronically on a display screen. There is etiquette for using a TTY. Only one person types at a time and when finished typing, the abbreviation GA (i.e., go ahead) is added to signal the other person that it is acceptable to respond. To conclude a call, the abbreviation SK (i.e., stop key) is used. After both callers type SK, or SKSK, the call is terminated. Today, with the proliferation of personal mobile phone and smartphone devices, there are many other ways to communicate. For those who would like to continue using their TTY hardware (select models may apply), it is possible to permit a mobile phone device to take the place of a hardwired landline connection by using an acoustic audio adapter patched into the mobile phone headphone jack.

The TTY can also be used to place calls to non-TTY users through the use of the Telecommunications Relay Service (TRS). This can work in one of two ways. First, the TTY user can place a call to the state's TTY number, which is typically 7-1-1, and give the phone number to be called to a relay operator. The relay operator has a TTY but will then place a speech-based call to the hearing person being called. Anything the TTY user says, the relay operator voices. Anything the hearing person says, the relay operator types back.

The same TTY etiquette applies here that was described earlier (e.g., the hearing caller verbally says, "Go Ahead"). Today, it is not necessary to have a desktop TTY. Anyone with Internet access can use one of several IP (Internet protocol) relay services (e.g., IP-Relay.com by Purple Communications and SprintIP.com). These IP relay services require registration to use them. It is also possible to use IP relay service technology with an app downloaded onto a mobile device (i.e., Apple iPad) with Internet access. It should be noted that the slow speed of a relay call can be frustrating for both parties, and the most successful relay calls are those when the individual with hearing loss keeps a positive attitude and advocates for all.

The second visual-based technology that comes to mind is a Voice-Carry Over (VCO) phone. A VCO call is a hybrid of the TTY call and a regular phone call. In this case, the individual with hearing loss may have speech that is well understood by others, but he or she cannot always understand the hearing person being called. Again, a relay operator serves in the same capacity by typing everything the hearing person says, but the individual with hearing loss will continue to use his or her own voice. In contrast to a TTY relay service call, a VCO may appear a little more natural, but the typing of the relay operator will lag slightly behind. Similar to the VCO, there are now specific captioned telephone companies (e.g., CapTel and CaptionCall) that offer relay services using proprietary phones that work just like regular acoustic phones using a landline connection, but also offer captioning through a high-speed Internet connection. Thus, both a telephone and Internet service are required.

A third, and final, visual-based technology is the use of video technology. Just as there are FaceTime and Skype video-based Internet and mobile phone communication tools, videophones (e.g., Sorenson nTouch and Purple Communications) are also available for those who communicate using sign language (Figure 10–3). Similar to the TTY, one videophone user can directly call another videophone user. Or, similar to a TTY relay call, a videophone user can call a hearing person. In this case, the relay operator is a trained sign language interpreter. Videophones use an Internet connection and webcam hardware, which must be professionally installed. Alternatively, videophone software for use on a computer and videophone apps for use on a mobile device may also be available.

Telecommunications Equipment Distribution Programs

In the United States, many states have a state-funded telecommunications equipment distribution program (TEDP) that provides free or low-cost telecommunication devices to qualified residents with disabilities. Although the requirements vary from state to state, in general, there is an application process for the individual with disability to indicate their state of residence, documented disability

(e.g., hearing loss, vision loss, or speech impairment), and documented financial need. For individuals with hearing loss, the types of telecommunications devices and accessories that might be available include, for example, TTY/TDD, amplified telephone, CapTel phone, talking phone, telephone alerting devices, and mobile phones. Individual TEDPs may partner with mobile service providers to offer special plans such as text-only (SMS; short message service) mobile plans. Readers are encouraged to visit the Telecommunications Equipment Distribution Program Association (TEDPA) website (http://www.tedpa.org/) to determine if their home state has a TEDP and to determine what the application requirements are as well as the types of telecommunication devices available from that program.

Summary

In this chapter, we covered a variety of ways that individuals with hearing loss can communicate by phone. It should be apparent now that we have largely moved away from hardwired, landline phones to mobile and Internet methods of telecommunication. For those who continue to prefer hardwired phones, there are a number of amplified phones on the market that help with both auditory and visual enhancements. Many mobile phones, and hearing aids, may have microphone (M) and telecoil (T) ratings to enhance the user's experience. A rating of at least M3/T3 or higher is best. Using a TTY or

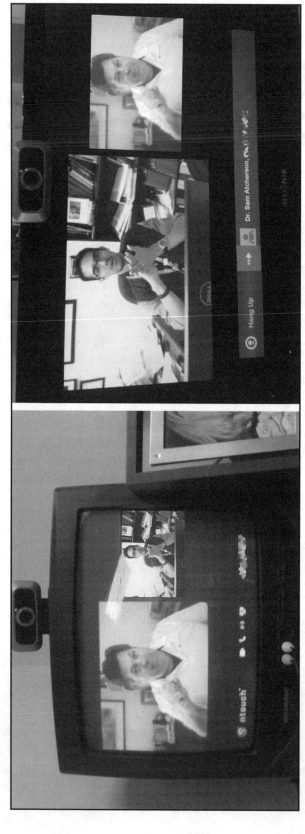

Figure 10–3. Example videoconference call using Sorensen nTouch via Internet connection. Sorenson performs professional installation of a webcam and router system at an agreed upon scheduled time (television is not included). In the left picture, the smaller image represents the person (*black vest*) who placed the call to another videophone user (*white shirt*). In the right picture, the smaller image represents the same person who received the call (*white shirt*). The entire conversation is carried out through sign language. Photo credit: Samuel R. Atcherson, PhD (*left*) and Timothy Lowe (*right*).

videophone, users can call another individual with the same technology to communicate via text or sign language. TTY, VCO, and related captioned phones all use relay operators to facilitate communication between the individual with hearing loss and the conversation partner. For the TTY, the relay operator will receive speech-based messages and translate that to text for the individual with hearing loss. VCO and captioned phones (CapTel and CaptionCall phones), which still use a relay operator, may provide a more natural phone conversation flow by allowing the individual to use his or her own voice. Some of these technologies may have already moved to mobile phone, tablet, and computer-based methods with appropriate mobile and/or Internet service. Finally, individuals with hearing loss could inquire with their state TEDP to find out if they may qualify for a free or greatly reduced in price phone aimed at equalizing telecommunications access for all citizens.

11

Text-Based Access Technologies[1]

Overview

This chapter draws attention to some powerful text-based access technologies that help facilitate communication in digital print form through the translation of speech-to-text and from text-to-text. These technologies are in contrast to text-to-speech (i.e., speech synthesis) which may help individuals unable to speak, and speech-to-speech which may offer some form of translation from one language to another. Deaf and hard of hearing people make up a diverse group with wide variation in type and severity of hearing loss, age at onset, communication modalities,

educational background, use of hearing aids or implant devices, and availability and accessibility of services. At extremes, some individuals have good ability to understand speech while listening and reading lips (also called speechreading), whereas others have great difficulty with both. It cannot be assumed that all deaf and hard of hearing individuals (including hearing individuals) are able to understand everything they hear even with optimized technology, nor can it be assumed that all have the ability to read lips or even be trained to read lips. For example, there are some Deaf individuals who do not use hearing-based technology (e.g., hearing aids or implantable

[1]Portions of this chapter are reprinted or modified from a previously published article by Atcherson, S. R., & Smith, R. E. (2010). I see what you're saying. *Hearing Health*, *26*, 30–34. Permission of Hearing Health Foundation.

devices) but have become quite adept at lipreading, whereas there are others who struggle with lipreading. Similarly, there are some individuals who use hearing-based technology who greatly benefit from lipreading, while there are others who do not. Taken further, there are some Deaf individuals who do not speak and will use sign language or text-based technology to communicate. The point of the foregoing discussion is to recognize that communication is a two-way street and existing technology can aid in facilitating two-way communication. In other situations, information may only need to be conveyed and could be available both acoustically through speech and visually through text.

The use of text to improve the capture of spoken language is not new. However, the method by which spoken language is converted to text has expanded from having professionals caption or transcribe live programming to having prescripted text-based files and sophisticated automatic speech recognition (ASR) technology. On most televisions today, the most common and well-recognized speech-to-text technology is closed captioning (CC). That is, once activated on a television (e.g., CC1), the dialogue or script from television shows, news sources, and advertisements shows up as white text on black bars. Similar technology has made its way into the entertainment and social media industry such as via Web-based videos (e.g., YouTube), digital video discs (DVD), Blu-ray discs (BD), and video streaming technology (e.g., Netflix and Hulu). Sometimes the captions are referred to as *subtitles* whose text may be available in more than one language.

In contrast to CC and subtitles, many may not be aware of other speech-to-text technology used in the classroom and in professional meetings. This type of technology is used not only for informational and educational purposes, but also to help facilitate dialogue among one or more individuals within that setting. Thus, anyone with hearing loss can benefit from reading what has been said, and by whom. A more recent development is the use of wearable automatic speech recognition (ASR) devices to aid in face-to-face communication. Many people today are quite familiar with various text-to-text technologies, such as text messaging via cellular short message service (SMS) and instant messaging (IM) through e-mail and social media sites. However, there are additional text-to-text technologies that may not have been considered to enable communication in educational situations, private sessions, and public areas.

This chapter is a broad one, which covers the various types of speech-to-text technologies and lesser known text-to-text technologies. A large portion of this chapter focuses on CC technology from which many other forms of speech-to-text technology have been based or inspired. This is particularly true for Web-based applications. In the United States, there is a rich technical, political, and entertainment history regarding the use of captioning that will be worthwhile reading. Throughout this chapter, we also showcase a few of the technologies currently available.

Closed Captioning

Today, more television programming than ever before is available with captioning in which the dialog appears as text on the screen, along with words to convey audible events such as music, laughter, and sound effects. Captioning used on television and in films can be beneficial to individuals who are deaf or hard of hearing, people learning English, and viewers in areas with high background noise. Captioning for recorded television programming was first developed in the early 1970s and over the course of the next decade was expanded to include live television events. Since the 1980s, the U.S. Congress has passed several laws improving the availability and required uses of captioning. These laws include the Television Decoder Circuitry Act of 1990, the Americans with Disabilities Act of 1990, the Telecommunications Act of 1996, and the Twenty-first Century Communication and Video Accessibility Act of 2010. These laws, combined with an increase in voluntary captioning, have helped foster an explosion of captioning accessibility. However, not all programming and venues are captioned, and consumer groups and others are continuing to push for captioning accessibility.

Captioning Basics

Captioning is transcribing or translating sound, whether that sound is spoken words, music, music with lyrics, or sound effects, into written text. Captions can be *open* or *closed*; open captions are always visible on a screen, while closed captions are embedded in the broadcast signal and must be accessed with dedicated equipment to be seen. Captions can be added to prerecorded video such as television programs and movies. Captioning can also occur during live events, such as a face-to-face workshop, conference, television newscast, or sporting event on television, with the use of Communication Access Realtime Translation (CART). Making the spoken word available as text immediately through CART developed out of the court reporting industry. The purpose of court reporting and CARTing, insofar as is possible, is to type a verbatim transcript of speech at various events, for example a deposition, conference speech, or class. A verbatim transcript is possible because this typing is performed on a shorthand machine, called a stenotype, that has 22 keys, including numbers (Figure 11–1). The CART writer depresses one or more keys simultaneously which documents the speech sounds being uttered. A software package converts that shorthand phonetic representation to text in real time through an internal dictionary. A person who is trained as a captioner or CART writer must type at least 180 words per minute with high accuracy, and many individuals can type 200 to 225 words per minute. As is seen later, CART is one of several captioning services available.

Many entities across the country offer the service of adding captions to preexisting video. The Described and Captioned Media Program maintains a list

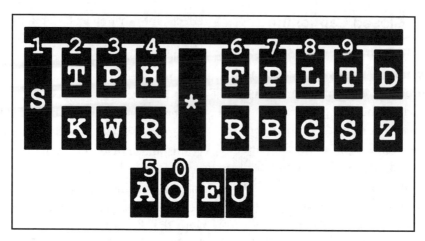

Figure 11–1. A stenotype keyboard.

of caption providers both in the United States and worldwide (http://www.dcmp.org/ai/10/).

Since its appearance in 1972, captioning for programs broadcast on television has been regulated by the Federal Communication Commission (FCC). Captioning regulation of Internet video such as news programs, streaming video, YouTube, and programming that was previously shown on television (e.g., Netflix, Hulu) has taken a few years to sort out. FCC rules promulgated in 2014 have helped the industry understand what types of videos must be captioned for the Web and who is responsible for adding those captions.

History of Captioning in the United States

The first captions in the United States were made in the late 1950s by Captioned Films for the Deaf. This organization was a forerunner of the Described and Captioned Media Program, a program currently funded by the U.S. Department of Education and administered by the National Association of the Deaf. The public first saw broadcast captions in 1971 at the *First National Conference on Television for the Hearing Impaired* in Knoxville, Tennessee, followed by a second demonstration of captioning at Gallaudet University, Washington, DC, in early 1972. These successful demonstrations led the U.S. Department of Health, Education, and Welfare's Office of Education, Bureau of Education for the Handicapped to fund research by the Public Broadcasting Service to further develop a captioning system. Open captioning, in which text is always visible on the screen, first appeared on television in 1972 on WGBH-Boston's *The French Chef* program with Julia Child. Closed captioning, text accessible only with a dedicated piece of equipment called a decoder, was first shown with the television program

The Mod Squad during its normal broadcast in the mid-1970s. Once closed captioning appeared, the FCC set aside *line 21* of the vertical blanking interval in the analog television signal, the only type of signal then available, as the closed caption transmission line. The Public Broadcasting Service, working with television networks debuted closed captioning in 1980 with the Sunday Night Movie on ABC, *Disney's Wonderful World* on NBC, and *Masterpiece Theatre* on PBS. IBM holds the distinction of having the first closed captioned television commercial. These closed and open captions gave access of prerecorded TV programming to individuals who were deaf or hard of hearing, but there was still no access to live TV events. Real-time, or live, captioning was developed by the National Captioning Institute and debuted on network television with the 1981 Sugar Bowl.

FCC regulations for captioning television programming began in earnest in 1993, following passage of the National Decoder Circuitry Act (1990) with the latest rules adopted in February 2014. These new guidelines (FCC, 2014) became effective on April 30, 2014, and specify, for the first time, quality standards for captioning:

- *Accurate:* Captions must match the spoken words in the dialogue and convey background noises and other sounds to the fullest extent possible.
- *Synchronous:* Captions must coincide with their corresponding spoken words and sounds to the greatest extent possible and must be displayed on the screen at a speed that can be read by viewers.
- *Complete:* Captions must run from the beginning to the end of the program to the fullest extent possible.
- *Properly placed:* Captions should not block other important visual content on the screen, overlap one another, or run off the edge of the video screen.

The FCC rules define live, near-live, and prerecorded programming. Live programming is broadcast simultaneously as it happens, near-live is broadcast within 24 hours of being recorded, and prerecorded is everything else. The rules also explain how the new standards apply to each type of programming and recognize that live and near-live programming present some difficulties with meeting the standards. The completeness of a program may be problematic because live captioning is slightly delayed from the actual program, and accuracy with live captioning can suffer because there is no time to review the captioning before sending it with the video signal.

Laws Governing Captioning

It may seem unnecessary to include information about the laws that govern captioning. However, in many instances the spread of captioning to different media types and different venues is driven by lawsuits. Thus, being familiar with the various laws that impact captioning availability is important for consumers and professionals alike.

The Television Decoder Circuitry Act of 1990 mandates that analog televisions and television circuitry equipped computers with picture screens of at least 13″ have the technology to decode closed captioning built into the device. Also included are digital television sets with a vertical screen measure of at least 7.8″, and stand-alone digital television tuners and boxes which access cable, satellite, and any other subscription television services, no matter the size of the viewing screen. This Act also empowers the FCC to ensure closed captioning remains available whenever new video technology is introduced.

The Americans with Disabilities Act of 1990 (ADA) and its 2008 amendments are important not for any technical aspects of captioning but for defining what venues (e.g., movie theaters, public stadiums) and companies (e.g., Netflix) are responsible for providing captioning with their programming. For example, the National Association for the Deaf (NAD) and others sued Netflix in 2010. These plaintiffs stated that Netflix did not have captions available in their "Watch Instantly" section. Because captions were not available there, they argued that Netflix practiced disability-based discrimination in providing their goods and services and were violating Title III of the ADA. When Netflix added Internet streaming to their business model, it had fundamentally changed how home entertainment programming was delivered, from physical discs (e.g., DVD and BD) to Internet streaming. The physical discs were likely to have captioning, whereas the Internet streaming did not, given the new technologies and formats being used. The lawsuit ended with a consent decree in October 2012, in which Netflix agreed to provide captioning within seven days of a program without captions launched on the Watch Instantly site by October 2016. The landmark ruling in the Netflix case provides two important points: (1) online video accessibility cannot be ignored any longer, legally covered by the ADA law; and (2) ruling that an online company's service (video streaming) is a "place of public accommodation" could extend the ADA's jurisdiction to any organization that publishes video (3PlayMedia, 2013) and not only brick and mortar companies. The Greater Los Angeles Agency on Deafness sued Time Warner (specifically Cable News Network or CNN) in 2013, in a lawsuit similar to the Netflix case, because CNN's streaming video on the Internet was not captioned. CNN argued that requiring the video captions violated CNN's right to free speech. The lower court ruled against CNN, stating that there was no objection to the content of CNN's video, only how it was conveyed to the public. Following the FCC's final rule published in August, 2014 that all video clips on the Internet must be captioned, CNN has had its appeal dismissed and has stated it will comply with that rule (Association of Southern California Defense Counsel, 2014).

The Telecommunications Act of 1996 was the first significant makeover of the Communications Act of 1934 in

62 years. One aspect of this law was that digital televisions with viewing screens of 13″ or more had to have built-in decoders for closed captions. A second outcome was the inclusion of the Internet in the FCC's decisions about broadcasting and frequency spectrum/bandwidth allotment. In addition, Title III, section 305 specifically addressed video programming accessibility. This section directed the FCC to perform an inventory of sorts, to determine how much video programming was closed captioned, how large the programming provider and owner were that provided the closed captioning, and several other pieces of data. This information served as baseline data for subsequent rules and regulations the FCC promulgated regarding who was responsible to provide captioning for programming.

The Twenty-First Century Communication and Video Accessibility Act of 2010 ensures that accessibility laws passed during the 1980s and 1990s will be updated to 21st century communications technologies. This law (1) requires video programs first shown with captions on television to have captions when shown on the Internet; (2) expands the caption requirement to devices that have screens smaller than 13″ (e.g., tablets, mobile smartphones); and (3) requires "video programming apparatuses," which include, for example, DVDs, Blu-ray players and software such as a streaming video player, to also record and play back captions that can be turned on and off. The FCC has stated there are some types of videos on the Web that do not require captioning: (1) consumer-generated media, for example, homemade movies, uploaded

to the Web; (2) Internet-only movies that were never aired on television; and (3) public, educational, and government access television.

In the 2010 National Association for the Deaf law-suit against Netflix mentioned previously, Netflix argued that the NAD lawsuit should be filed under the CVAA legislation rather than the ADA; that was significant because at the time captioning was not mentioned in the CVAA legislation. The judge ruled that these two laws were not mutually exclusive, which allowed the suit to move forward. It was at that point that Netflix decided to settle out of court.

Captioning in Different Media and Venues

Prerecorded Programs

The process for adding captions to prerecorded programs, known as *offline captioning*, has undergone dramatic change in the past 30 years, owing mainly to the switch from analog to digital technologies. In the past, captioning has been time intensive, for example, one hour of programming might take 10 hours to caption. Recent advances in computer technology and software, however, have resulted in offline captioning becoming much faster although the basic steps remain similar.

Offline captioning is done once a broadcast program has completed postproduction but prior to airing. The content producer, distributor, or broadcaster provides a digital copy of the program to a captioning vendor. The digital copy can be a video file or DVD and must include a time code that matches the master program copy. The captioning vendor will check this copy for sequential and error-free time codes, usable audio, and sufficient video quality. This evaluation is important to identify any problems that could slow the captioning process and allows the captioning vendor personnel to work with the producer to fix any issues. If the captioning vendor does not receive a verbatim transcript from the producer, the next step is to generate a transcript that includes not only dialog but also sound effects, music notations, and any other nonverbal features. Once a transcript is available, the actual captioning is done. Captioning consists of the text being separated into individual captions, for example, speaker by speaker or a particular sound effect, positioning the captions at the appropriate locations on the screen, and associating each caption with the exact time and duration it should appear. Once the captioning process is completed, captioning vendor personnel will review the newly made file for accuracy, spelling, timing, and overall quality. The final step the captioning vendor undertakes is to *encode*, which is combining the caption file with the submitted video file. The final product, the encoded submaster, can be returned to the producer via e-mail, file transfer protocol, or whatever media the client prefers.

Captioning for a broadcast program can appear on the screen in a few different ways. First, *pop-on* captions are one to two lines of text that are visible for a few seconds then disappear. They can be placed anywhere on the screen, making them

quite useful to indicate that a nonspeech sound, such as a school bell, occurred off screen or away from the main action. *Roll-up* captions (Figure 11–2) are typically a match to the spoken word and synchronized to the speaker. Greater-than symbols (>>) indicate a different speaker. Each line rolls up and then disappears from the screen as an entire, new bottom line appears. *Paint-on* captions are similar to roll-up captions; they are verbatim with the spoken word. The main difference from roll-up captions is that paint-on appear from left to right, not all at once.

Live Events

Historically, the FCC has allowed national and local news broadcasters to convert teleprompter script into captions. Naturally this enabled viewers who are deaf and hard of hearing access to those portions of news programs with that scripted information but did not provide access for portions without scripting. Under the 2014 regulations, news broadcasters are now allowed to script more of their news shows, including sports, weather, and late-breaking stories. The new rules require that portions of these programs which cannot be pre-scripted be made accessible through a "crawl" across the bottom portion of the screen.

Other live programs, such as sporting events and awards programs, and programs streamed on the Internet, use "real-time captioning." Real-time captioning is captions being added as the event is being video and audio recorded. The captioner may be at the location of

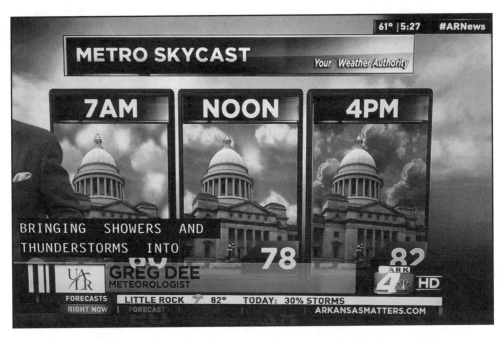

Figure 11–2. Television captioning (*lower left*) of the weather in Arkansas on a news station.

the event or performing the captioning remotely. Generally with real-time captioning, the text is seen in two to three lines and may be either open or closed. Just as with offline captioning, real-time captions can be displayed on any type of video screen, including televisions, monitors, film screens, or the Web.

Real-time captions can be added via typing (see CART section) or voice writing. Voice writing converts speech to text in real time and is a different method used to make the spoken word available visually. Voice writers use speech recognition software such as *Dragon*, combined with CART software, such as *Eclipse*CAT. According to Dessa Van Schuyver (personal communication, 2014), owner of the Real Time Voice Academy, *Dragon*

software is highly accurate at speaking rates up to about 190 words per minute. Because captioners are able to type upwards of 200 to 225 words per minute, these two methods of captioning are similar in the time needed to provide the captions.

Cinema

Under the ADA, movie theaters have long been required to provide hearing assistive technology for patrons, but they have not had to provide any particular type of device(s); induction loops, infrared devices, FM systems, and captioning all met the letter of the law. In most cases, however, providing captioned movies had not been possible or been expensive for theater owners to do. Two events have occurred recently that have changed that situation: the introduction of digital movie projection capabilities and a court ruling. In the case *State of Arizona v. Harkins Amusement Enterprises* (2010), the Ninth Circuit Court of Appeals ruled that movie theaters must show close-captioned movies unless that results in a "fundamental alteration" or an "undue burden" to the business. The second event has been the development and spread of digital cinema. Digital cinema was introduced in 1998 in the United States. In 2002 several motion picture studios formed the *Digital Cinema Initiatives* to set standards for this format. Digital cinema technology is computer based; theaters receive the movies on a computer hard drive or via satellite or fiber-optic broadband and must load the file(s) onto the server of the theater projection system. The important point for closed captioning is that the captions are stored in a separate digital channel and not directly on the 35-mm film, as was the case with analog movies. The advent of 3D movies in the same time frame likely provided encouragement to the larger theater chains to replace the 35-mm projection systems with this newer digital technology, making the availability of captioning to patrons more manageable for theaters.

There are a variety of ways and devices to display movie dialog as text in a theater. The most familiar is probably subtitles, when the English text is displayed at the bottom of the screen for movies made in other languages. Subtitles are essentially open captions, visible to the whole audience throughout the program. In fact, several countries (e.g., England and Spain) use the term *subtitle* to refer to all captions on television, movies, and so forth, and call the captions discussed in this chapter "subtitles for the deaf and hard of hearing." In the United States, few movies are released with open captions with the trend toward closed captions accessible to individual patrons using some type of dedicated device.

The earliest device developed to provide access to closed captions in movies is the Rear Window Captioning System, developed by WGBH-Boston and artist Rufus Butler Seder. The Rear Window system consists of a light-emitting diode text display board mounted at the rear of the theater. The text on this display is reversed. Patrons desiring access to the captions are given clear acrylic panels that attach to their seats and are adjustable, allowing the patron to sit anywhere in the theater. These panels reflect the captions displayed at the back of the room, superimposing the captions across the bottom of the movie screen to read correctly. Thus, only the patrons with acrylic panels see the captions.

The Rear Window Captioning System (Figure 11–3) was first seen in a commercial cinema in November 1997 in Sherman Oaks, California, with the Universal Picture film, *The Jackal*. WGBH, a public broadcasting nonprofit company in Boston, Massachusetts, collaborated with General Cinema Theatres, Universal Pictures, and Digital Theater Systems, to bring this captioning system to the public. In addition to commercial cinemas, the Rear Window system is available in

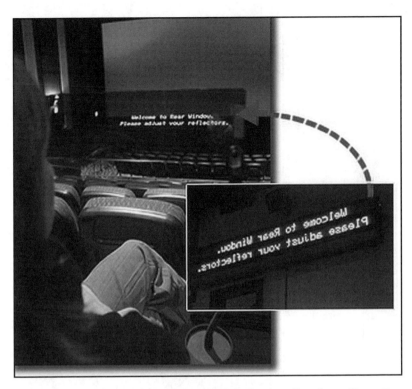

Figure 11–3. Rear Window Captioning System "backward" caption text display on the back wall (*right*) that is sent in readable format to reflective acrylic panel in front of the patron (*left*). Image courtesy of WGBH Educational Foundation.

some IMAX theaters, National Park Visitor Centers, and Disney Theme Parks and Resorts. As of 2010, the last year for which there are records, about 300 theaters in the United States were using the Rear Window system (Peter Villa, WGBH, personal communication, 2014).

Doremi Labs, a technology company specializing in digital cinema and broadcast products, introduced the CaptiView Display closed captioning device (Figure 11–4) for movie theaters in 2010. The Doremi device fits into the cup holder of any theater seat and uses a Wi-Fi signal to receive encrypted closed captions. The captions display on three lines. Used with the CaptiView Transmitter (a USB device) and the CaptiView software package, the CaptiView system has a range of 262 feet (80 meters), enabling patrons to sit anywhere in the theater. The Doremi system also communicates via Ethernet with the Rear Window Captioning System and establishes a connection while sending time code and text files so they are displayed on the Rear Window panels in sync with the image (Jesus Alvarado, Doremi Labs, personal communication, 2014).

Sony Corporation has entered the accessibility realm for movie theaters

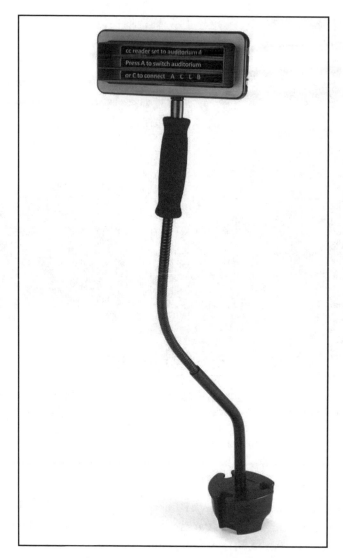

Figure 11–4. CaptiView Display closed caption receiver for movie theaters. Image courtesy of Doremi Labs.

with their Sony Entertainment Access Glasses (Figure 11–5). The captions are holographically displayed, appear to float "in the air," and are bright and easy to read. These glasses are synchronized with the theater's digital projection system through a wireless receiver. Both neck-loops and headphones can be plugged into the receiver to increase the volume for assisted listening. The Entertainment Access Glasses can be worn alone or over one's prescription glasses for both 2D and 3D movies (with an added polarized filter).

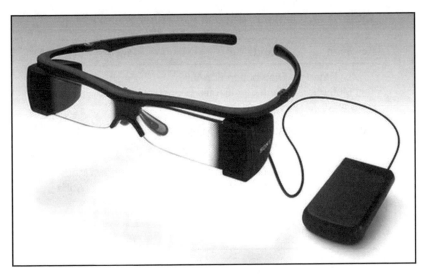

Figure 11–5. Sony's Entertainment Access Glasses with Audio (STW-C140GI) and receiver box. Image courtesy of Sony Corporation.

Captioning on the Web

As explained earlier, the CVAA of 2010 requires programs shown over broadcast media that had captions (and at the time of this writing in 2014 includes most broadcast programming) also have captions when replayed on the Web. In addition, clips or short portions of programs shown on the Web must have captions. Just as with broadcast programming, Internet program captioning can be added post-production or live.

This mandate would appear to be somewhat simple to accomplish. Most broadcast programs already have captions and therefore do not need any further work to be shown on the Web with captions. The reality is quite a bit more complicated, however. The complexity arises from the many formats and platforms that various companies have developed over the years that can be used for video and audio uploaded to the Web. Just as with broadcast programming, the captioning information must be encoded and added to/conjoined with the video and must be encoded for the particular player used, for example, Windows Media Player, QuickTime, or Flash. In addition to the encoding file being different based on the player, the Web video can be in different formats; three of the most common ones at present are H.264, MPEG-4, and FlashVP6. There are caption editing programs that generate the encoded file, which essentially combines the program transcript with the timing information. The various players also have encoded file specifications, some of which are proprietary while others use general file standards. Table 11–1 lists some of the most common formats in use and which players those work with.

Table 11–1. Common Caption File Formats and Players

Acronym	Stands for	Players
TTML (Timed Text Markup Language)	Distribution Format Exchange Profile	Flash, YouTube
SMIL	Synchronized Multimedia Integration Language	Quicktime, RealPlayer
SAMI	Synchronized Accessible Media Interchange	Windows Media Player, YouTube
SRT	SubRip	YouTube
SUB	SubViewer	YouTube

Google, owner and operator of YouTube, has as its mission to make all Internet information universally accessible. As part of that mission, the YouTube captioning team offers a platform that allows anyone to upload already-created captions in 20-plus different formats. Furthermore, all of those captions can be displayed on all YouTube players. YouTube's captioning team has also built automated captioning that uses speech recognition technology along with a transcript file to time and place the captions (Ellis, Miller, Daniali, & McCarty, 2014). Although speech recognition technology has improved over the last few years, any additional sounds on an audio track (e.g., background noise, music to accompany the video) that overlap the speech will decrease the accuracy of these automated captions.

There also exist other Web- and computer-based captioning programs. Web-based programs are often free, accept a variety of file formats, and may allow you to export your product in a standard caption file such as those listed in Table 11–1. Disadvantages of Web-based programs are that (1) one may not be able to save the work and return to it, (2) the captioned video must be available via a public URL, or (3) you may have to access your captioned file through a third-party URL. Computer-based software has advantages (including output to a file and the ability to work offline) and disadvantages (may be platform specific, more technical skill needed, only proprietary file formats available). If the video program owners and distributors decide to incorporate captioning into their production process, SoftDoc, Inc., has a hardware plus software solution for which they offer software updates and device replacement as needed (personal communication, SoftDoc, Inc., 2014). The decision of which technologies to use must rest with the captioners and their needs.

The FCC has set rules that Web captions have to be at least as good as television captions, and that the end user must have control over the following: font size, font style, character color, opacity, edge attributes, caption background, language selection, and preview/setting retention. Because there are many available caption formats, the FCC adopted the Society of Motion Picture and Television Engineers Timed Text (SMPTE-TT) caption format as a "safe harbor interchange and delivery format." Therefore, if video is captioned in the SMPTE-TT style, that captioning meets the FCC requirements, although other formats also meet those requirements.

The complexity of captioning for the Web exists currently for a variety of reasons. These include the newness of the FCC rules and regulations mandating the captioning; the multiplicity of software platforms; proprietary versus general file types; and whether to use automated speech recognition captioning software, use Web-based programs, or add captions via an in-house computer-based program. As has happened with other technological advances, these alternatives will likely coalesce around fewer, more standardized options, thus making the captioning of Web video commonplace.

Speech-to-Text Technology in the Classroom and Meetings

A major obstacle for students and meeting participants with hearing loss is having complete access to auditory information presented. Access to auditory information is largely limited because the environ-ment can be noisy, especially in classrooms with young fidgety children and in group settings with active dialogue. This extra noise makes it difficult to hear any one particular person over the noise. Hearing assistive technology (see Chapters 6 through 9) may be helpful to overcome the effect of noise and to improve the signal-to-noise ratio (SNR) of desired speech. However, if the individual with hearing loss still depends heavily on lip-reading or speechreading, the auditory information may only be of limited help. If the principal speaker (e.g., teacher, presenter, or facilitator) engages learners and participants by moving around the room, there will be times that visual access to the face and mouth will be lost. Finally, students and meeting participants who would like to take their own notes are at a disadvantage, because as soon as they shift their attention to write something, they will have already missed potentially critical points being made by the speaker. In the classroom or comparable meeting environment, the captioned information is transcribed and displayed on a projector screen or laptop display so that individuals with hearing loss can read the information as it is being presented with a very short lag time. Figure 11–6 shows one example of the speech-to-text technology used in a classroom setting.

Speech-to-text services are generally categorized into three broad groups: steno-based CART, text interpreting (C-Print or TypeWell), and automatic speech recognition (ASR). Each of these technologies requires a specially trained professional who knows how to properly

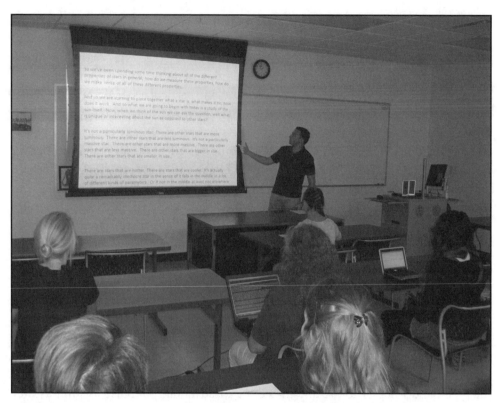

Figure 11–6. An example of text interpreting for a student with hearing loss in a classroom setting. The instructor takes his usual position in front of the classroom where he interacts with the entire class. In a strategic location that is not disruptive to other students in the classroom, the speech-to-text provider (*near center*) uses a laptop computer to transcribe the lecture. The student with hearing loss on the far right is able to read the lecture in "real time." Photo credit: Kathleen Becker.

set up and operate the software and equipment. CART and text interpreting services involve listening and typing, while ASR involves listening and speaking. These professionals undergo many hours of training and practice to develop and improve their efficiency and accuracy in listening and typing (or listening and speaking) at the same time for somewhat long durations of time. For long classes or meetings, there may be two providers who work in teams offering each other breaks at regular intervals. Regardless of the technology, students and meeting participants may have access to an electronic or paper copy of the entire session as it was produced. Clients can ask for copies ahead of time. Additionally, most, if not all, of these services can be provided remotely so long as the provider is able to hear what is happening in the room. That is, an arrangement can be made for the service to be provided without the provider's physical presence. Where there are many similarities in speech-to-text services, there are also many differences. Below is a brief discussion of each technology, and Table 11–2 shows some of these similarities and differences in the text output.

Table 11–2. Attributes and Output Examples of Three Different Types of Speech-to-Text Services

Service	Attributes	Output Example
CART	Verbatim-ness: High Accuracy: High Number of pages: ~15–20 Typing using a special keyboard	Teacher: I forgot my textbook in the office. Oh, wait a minute. No, I have it here. Okay, let's get started now. This science experiment can be done in Australia, Europe, or South America and the result is always the same because the elements are the same. Display: I FORGOT MY TEXTBOOK IN THE OFFICE. OH, WAIT A MINUTE. NO, I HAVE IT HERE. OKAY, LET'S GET STARTED. THIS SCIENCE EXPERIMENT CAN BE DONE IN AUSTRALIA, EUROPE, OR SOUTH AMERICA AND THE RESULT IS ALWAYS THE SAME BECAUSE THE ELEMENTS ARE THE SAME.
C-Print/ Typewell	Verbatim-ness: Medium to High Accuracy: High Number of pages: ~6–10 Typing using a laptop computer	Teacher: This science experiment can be done in Australia, Europe, or South America and the result is always the same because the elements are exactly the same. Display: THIS SCIENCE EXPERIMENT CAN BE DONE ANYWHERE IN THE WORLD AND THE RESULT WILL ALWAYS BE THE SAME BECAUSE THE ELEMENTS ARE EXACTLY THE SAME.
Automatic Speech Recognition	Verbatim-ness: High Accuracy: Medium to High Number of pages: ~15–20 Speaking into a special mask with built-in microphone	Teacher: Good morning! Are you ready to learn about the history of this great nation? Let's start with the Civil War. Display: COULD MORNING! ARE YOU READY TO LEARN ABOUT THE HISTORY OF DISCRIMINATION? LETTUCE START WITH THE CIVIL WAR.

Source: Table reprinted with permission by *Hearing Health Magazine.*

CART involves the use of a stenograph or stenotype machine. Unlike the traditional computer keyboard, stenographs have two rows of keys without markings (recall Figure 11–1). Rather than typing each word exactly as it is spelled, the provider uses a shorthand method in which various keys are pressed in particular clusters to construct each word. CART is often credited for being verbatim. That is, every word that is spoken, regardless of relevance to the lecture, is captured and typed. A potential disadvantage, however, is that a lecture may produce as many as 20 pages of paper or more.

With text interpreting (C-Print and TypeWell), the provider uses a laptop computer and a partial shorthand method. Although all letter keys are available on laptop computer keyboards, abbreviations of common words are typically used to form whole words. Long words can often be written without the vowels and the software will select the closest word match possible and fill in the vowels. The output of this type of service typically uses a meaning-to-meaning approach, rather than a verbatim approach. Unlike CART where every word is transcribed, only the main points of the information are included and any repetitions and corrections that the teacher makes are not included. Text interpreting is similar to American Sign Language interpreting because the full meaning of the message is relayed without having to translate each word. Because of the meaning-to-meaning approach, a hard copy of the lecture will take up fewer pages than would be expected for CART. Certain special-

ized versions of C-Print and TypeWell are available that allow students a more interactive experience. For example, if the output of C-Print or TypeWell is projected to another laptop, then the student may have the option of adding his or her own notes, or deleting anything that he or she feels is irrelevant. Another recent feature is that students and meeting participants may receive C-Print and TypeWell transcriptions on a mobile device such as the iPhone, iPad, or Android-based device using an Internet connection (mobile cellular plan) or available Wi-Fi (Figure 11–7). If neither is available, TypeWell can still work by having the provider create a virtual access point to any Wi-Fi–enabled device such as an iPad.

Finally, ASR involves the provider speaking into a special mask with built-in microphone and everything he or she says is transcribed automatically by the computer software. Because of the speech recognition capabilities of the software, little to no typing is involved. For automatic speech recognition to work well, the software must be able to understand the provider's speech, and the provider must dictate as clearly as he or she can. Thus, the computer is "trained" and sets up a profile for that provider. Whenever the computer misunderstands a word, the provider can correct it "on the fly" or later. Like CART, automatic speech recognition is said to be verbatim.

In a school setting, the speech-to-text provider will "follow" the student to each of his or her classes where the service is needed. Thus, the provider is to be treated as a team member in the education and

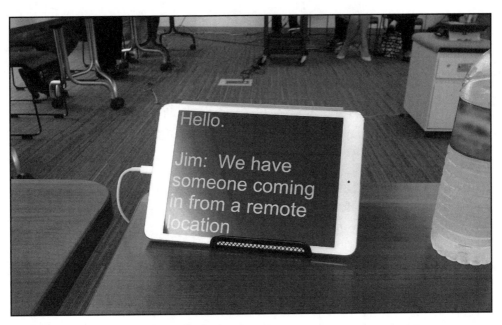

Figure 11–7. Example of the C-Print System on an iPad Mini used in a large meeting room. Photo credit: Samuel R. Atcherson, PhD.

advocacy of the student. However, the provider is not personally responsible for the welfare of the student, is typically not involved in educational decisions, and should not be used as a personal messenger to communicate with the student. The provider will use the time available between each class to set up and pack away his or her equipment for transport.

At meetings that draw large numbers of people with hearing loss, such as the annual Hearing Loss Association of America convention, it is not uncommon to find speech-to-text technologies at many of the sessions and workshops. The output of the speech-to-text service is prominently displayed on a large screen so that anyone in the audience is able to read the text.

Personal Speech-to-Text Technologies

The advent of mobile smartphone technology, wireless Bluetooth communication, and wearable wristband/watch systems has made available new assistive technology applications. For example, both Apple and Android-based smartphone devices have ASR technology. One company, Digital Army Devices (http://iseewhaty-ousay.com/), has taken advantage of that technology and developed a small handheld display device to transcribe what another person speaks into an Android-based smartphone. More recently, they have taken this technology further and created an app that pairs with the Pebble Watch (https://getpebble.com/) and the Android Wear (http://www.android.com/intl/en_us/wear/). As an example, to make this work on the Pebble Watch, the Android-device smartphone user must download the iseewhatyousay app from Google Play and from Pebble onto their smartphone and watch, respectively. The two apps are then loaded and synchronized. After synchronization, someone can speak into the built-in microphone on the smartphone and after a short time delay, the transcription would appear on the watch after a gentle vibration for the Pebble wearer. The obvious way to use this setup is for the person with hearing loss to wear the Pebble Watch and use his or her own smartphone as the microphone. The developers say that they are working on an Apple iOS-based app as well. Figure 11–8 shows an example of this wearable speech-to-text technology.

Text-to-Text Technology

Most individuals today with cellular service and Internet access are generally

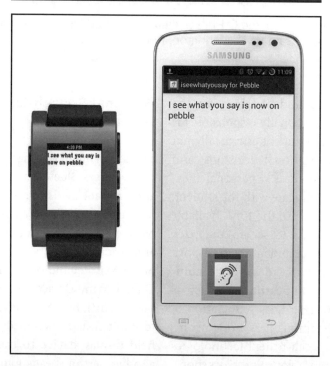

Figure 11–8. Example of a wearable speech-to-text technology in the form of a Pebble Watch synchronized with an Android-based smartphone using the iseewhatyousay app. Image courtesy of iseewhatyousay.com and Digital Army Devices.

familiar with text-to-text communication in the form of cellular-based text messages (short message service [SMS]) and Web-based instant messenging (IM). These services are enjoyed by individuals across the world, whether or not they have hearing loss. A more formal text-to-text experience is achievable using the SComm Ubiduo. The Ubiduo 2 is SComm's most recent hardware version, but it is a clever interlocking, dual-keyboard and display communication system that comes in a wired or wireless package. The two keyboards with text display fold together and can be carried like a laptop computer. The wireless version of the Ubiduo 2 uses the 2.4 GHz communication network system (previously described in Chapter 9) with an effective communication distance of up to 300 feet. No cellular or Wi-Fi connection is required. Such a system would be ideal for individuals with significant hearing loss or voice impairments. When a sign language interpreter cannot be secured, the Ubiduo 2 offers an attractive communication alternative that can be used anywhere. The only downside is that both communication partners must be able to type. Figure 11–9 shows an example of the Ubiduo 2 system.

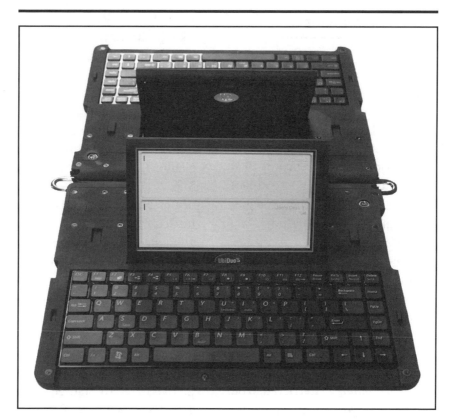

Figure 11–9. Ubiduo 2 from SComm, Inc. Image courtesy of SComm, Inc.

Summary

Speech-to-text services are a wonderful accommodation for people with hearing loss, and for those who communicate in other spoken languages. Each of the services described above is an attractive option for visual and readable access to spoken auditory information. Not only can the information be displayed in real time, but it can also be pre-scripted or post-captioned. Each service has its advantages and disadvantages, and none is perfect.

References

3PlayMedia. (2013). *How the ADA impacts online video accessibility.* Retrieved from http://info.3playmedia .com/rs/3playmedia/images/ADA-Brief.pdf

Americans with Disabilities Act of 1990, Pub. L. 101-336, 104 Stat. 327. (1990). Retrieved from http://www.gpo.gov/ fdsys/pkg/STATUTE-104/pdf/STAT UTE-104-Pg327.pdf

Association of Southern California Defense Counsel. (2014). *Verdict, 2.* Retrieved from http://www.ascdc.org/ PDF/ASCDC%2014-2.pdf

Consumer and Governmental Affairs Bureau. Federal Communications Commission. (n.d.). *Captioning of Internet video programming.* Retrieved from http://www.fcc.gov/guides/captioning-internet-video-programming

Consumer and Governmental Affairs Bureau. Federal Communications Commission. (2014). *Closed captioning on television.* Retrieved from http://www .fcc.gov/guides/closed-captioning

Described and Captioned Media Program. (2011). *Captioning key.* National Association for the Deaf. Retrieved from http://www.dcmp.org/captioningkey/

Ellis, B., Miller, J., Daniali, A., & McCarty, B. (2014). *Best practices for implementing accessible video captioning.* Huntington Beach, CA: Streaming Media West. Retrieved from http://www.3play media.com/2014/01/10/future-acces sibility-video-captions-according-google-youtube/?mkt_tok=3RkMMJ WWfF9wsRokva3IZKXonjHpfsX56u wkWK%2BwlMI%2F0ER3fOvrPUfGj I4DTMJqI%2BSLDwEYGJlv6SgFTbT BMbVk1bgLUhY%3D

Federal Communications Commission. (n.d.). *What we do.* Retrieved from http://www.fcc.gov/what-we-do

National Association of the Deaf, et al. v. Netflix, Case No. 3:11-cv-30168. (F.D. MA, 2011).

Office of Public Affairs. Department of Justice. (2014). *Justice Department announces proposed amendment to Americans with Disabilities Act regulations to expand access to movie theaters for individuals with hearing and vision disabilities.* Retrieved from http:// www.justice.gov/opa/pr/2014/July/14-crt-781.html

Telecommunications Act of 1996, Pub. L. 104-104, 110 Stat. 56, codified at 47 U.S.C. §609 note. Retrieved from http://www.gpo.gov/fdsys/pkg/PLAW-

104publ104/html/PLAW-104publ104.htm

Television Decoder Circuitry Act of 1990, Pub. L. 101-431, 104 Stat. 960, codified at 47 U.S.C. §609 note. Retrieved from http://transition.fcc.gov/Bureaus/OSEC/library/legislative_histories/1395.pdf

Twenty-First Century Communications and Video Accessibility Act of 2010, Pub. L. 111–260, 124 Stat. 2751, codified as amended at 47 U.S.C. §609 note. Retrieved from http://www.gpo.gov/fdsys/pkg/PLAW-111publ260/pdf/PLAW-111publ260.pdf

12

Alerting Devices and Services

Introduction

This chapter focuses on assistive technologies designed to signal (alert or prompt) individuals with hearing loss. Many signaling technologies may have been designed with hearing individuals in mind, yet they remain inaccessible for individuals with hearing loss (e.g., not loud enough).Fortunately, there are many different kinds of signaling technologies available for individuals with hearing loss that help to promote greater independence and quality of life, as well as to provide an indication that there is an event of importance or that there is an emergency. The manner in which individuals with hearing loss can be signaled will be in one or more forms involving the sensation of sound, light, and vibration. It would be difficult to organize this chapter based purely on each sensory method as many signalers today use a combination of the three. Instead, we organize this chapter based on the types of signaling technologies that serve specific purposes. Mobile phone tips are also discussed as appropriate to this chapter.

Alarm Clock

"How can I wake myself up in the morning?"

Alarm clocks are purposely designed to disturb sleep through the use of sound patterns that are intended to be irritating.

When the irritating sound pattern alone is not enough to arouse a person, sometimes making it louder (or progressively louder) is all that is needed. Generally speaking, the more severe the hearing loss, the less efficient sound will be, and the more likely light and vibration will be needed. In extreme situations, heavy sleepers with less severe hearing loss may benefit from the addition of light and vibration signaling from an alarm clock. Today, there are quite a few alarm clock signalers available that provide one or more sensory methods. For some individuals with hearing loss, a loud, sound-based alarm is all that is needed. Retail and online stores that sell standard alarm clocks may already have products designed for heavy sleepers, and they provide different sound alert patterns promising to wake even the heaviest sleepers. In the event that these products are not sufficiently loud, the individual with hearing loss may need to pursue an alarm clock through an assistive device store. Some of these assistive alarm clocks have sound outputs of 113 dB SPL. For reference, that is comparable to the intensity of a chainsaw. Figure 12–1 shows examples of hardwired and portable (travel) vibrating alarm clocks.

Alarm clocks that offer light and vibration sensations come in a variety of forms. For example, some alarm clocks have a receptacle that permits plugging in an ordinary bedside lamp. Others have built-in flashing light systems. In either case, the alarm clock will typically cause the light source to flash in a particular pattern, rather than simply turn the light source on. If light alone is enough to rouse a sleeper, a bedside lamp plugged into a simple electronic timer may be all that is needed. These electronic timers can be found in department and hard-

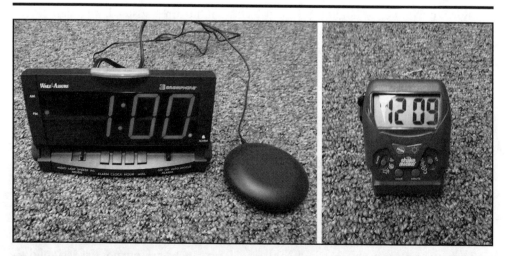

Figure 12–1. Examples of Ameriphone Wake Assure hardwired (*left*) and Shake Awake portable travel (*right*) alarm clocks. The hardwired alarm clock has an external bed vibrator connected to it, whereas the portable alarm clock has a built-in vibration motor. Photo credit: Samuel R. Atcherson, PhD.

ware stores to control light for security purposes, to save energy, or offer strict UV light regimens to growing plants. For vibration signaling, a large oscillating vibrator disc can typically be connected to an alarm clock signaler, which is then typically placed between the mattress and box spring. For most individuals, the durability of the vibrator is sufficiently strong. For heavy sleepers, an additional trick is to add a large piece of plywood in between the mattress and box springs so that when the vibrator goes off, the entire piece of plywood also vibrates as an effective accentuation. For others, both light and vibrator are best.

Mobile Phone Tip: Alarm Clock

Soon to be released, inventors Patrick Seypura and Alec Satterfly have developed Alarmify. Alarmify is an app and vibration device system synced together. The mobile phone serves as the clock, and when the alarm goes off, it triggers the motor in the vibrator. Seypura and Satterly are licensing the technology through another company, named Certify. Though not yet available, interested consumers can check for updates at http://cenify.com/product/alarmify/

Emergency Alerts

"I can't always hear fire and smoke detectors in my home, and I dread the day there is a severe natural disaster warning that I might miss!"

There are a variety of emergency alert signalers. Similar to standard fire, smoke, and carbon monoxide alarms seen in homes and offices, assistive emergency alert signalers will have enhanced or new features. For example, some of these products may feature louder than average signals (>90 dB) and may also have a flashing strobe light feature (Figure 12–2). Many of these products are wall mounted and powered either by battery or by electricity, although some are of the tabletop type. Some of these products serve as transmitters and will send alerts to a bed vibrator, or one of several compatible receivers. For example, the Bellman Visit Optical Smoke Alarm transmitter can send a signal to a vibrating alarm clock receiver, an audible receiver, and a vibrating pager receiver. It may be advantageous to have several products strategically placed around the home or office, or have a variety of receivers with the proper transmitting alert device.

Care should be taken to ensure that these emergency products for purchase meet certain standards. The National Fire Protection Association (NFPA) publishes a number of codes and standards. One such standard relevant to emergency products is NFPA 72 (National Fire Alarm and Signal Code), which covers the application, installation, location, performance, inspection, testing, and maintenance of fire alarm systems, supervising station alarm systems, public emergency alarm reporting systems, fire warning equipment and emergency communications systems (ECSs), and their components. The NFPA website lists several manufacturers, distributors, and retailers

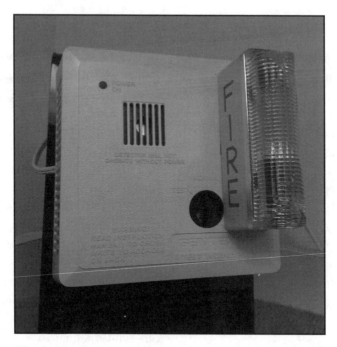

Figure 12–2. Example wall-mounted smoke alarm with photoelectric strobe light station and loud solid-state horn (~90 dB) by Gentex Corporation. Photo credit: Samuel R. Atcherson, PhD.

of smoke alarms for "people who are deaf or hard-of-hearing" that meet Underwriters Laboratories standard 1971 (UL 1971). Code UL 1971 (Signaling Devices for the Hearing Impaired) is one that is specific to individuals with hearing loss whose approved products are in accordance also with NFPA 72. ACE Hardware Corporation, BRK Electronics, Gentex Corporation, Kidde Fire Safety, and Menards, Inc., are all companies specifically listed by the NFPA at the writing of this book. As there may be products marketed that do not meet performance and evaluation standards, it is strongly recommended that consumers look for emergency products from one of the companies listed, with

clear indication that the product is UL 1971 approved. More importantly, these products should be marked "UL 1971 listed" indicating that they comply with applicable safety requirements and are listed in a published national directory.

For weather alerts, a National Weather Radio (NWR) receiver system can be acquired. There are two options: (1) adapter for deaf and hard of hearing to be used with a standard NWA receiver or (2) NWA receiver package designed specifically for individuals with hearing loss (e.g., Midland Weather Alert Radio transmitter with Silent Call Communications receivers). This alerting device can provide some of the same audible, light, and vibration alerts to various receivers whenever there are threats of tornadoes, hurricanes, floods, and other severe conditions. The weather bulletins will come from the National Ocean and Atmospheric Administration (NOAA). An example NWR is shown in Figure 12–3. More information about the specific NWR products designed to assist individuals with hearing loss can be found at http://www.nws.noaa.gov/nwr/info/special_needs.html

Mobile Phone Tip: Emergency Alerts

Rather than relying only on weather-related alerts from the television, radio, or community sirens, a mobile phone user can receive text (SMS; short message service) alerts wirelessly to his or her device. There are a number of different downloadable weather and/or emergency apps available for mobile phone consumers. The National Weather Service (NWS) does not send text messages (or e-mails) directly to the general public. However, there are a number of third-party services and the NWS has compiled a list of mobile apps that provide alerts (http://www.weather.gov/subscribe). It should be noted that the NWS does not directly endorse these apps. Rather, third-party providers and services request to be added to this list. NWS recommends that consumers have more than one way to receive alerts, including multiple apps, if necessary. For disaster-specific apps (e.g., hurricane, tornado, flood, earthquake, etc.), the American Red Cross also offers apps.

Another useful service is available for non-weather emergency alerts. The CTIA-The Wireless Association (http://www.ctia.org) along with the Federal Communications Commission (FCC) and the Federal Emergency Management Agency (FEMA), developed the Wireless Emergency Alerts (WEA) for mobile phones. WEA-capable mobile phones receive text-like messages for one of three different alerts: (1) presidential alerts issued by the president or designee, (2) imminent threat alerts for natural or man-made disasters, and (3) AMBER alerts for abducted children. Interested individuals should contact their wireless carriers to determine if their mobile phone is WEA-enabled and whether WEAs are provided in their area. On some mobile phones, WEA may need to be activated, and wireless consumers are not charged for these alerts. A list of participating wireless carriers can be found at http://www.ctia.org/your-wireless-life/consumer-tips/wireless-emergency-alerts

Sound Monitor and Motion Detectors

"I want to remain aware of my surroundings, and hate missing important text messages and phone calls."

There are hundreds of different products on the market to help individuals with hearing loss stay alert to a variety of environmental cues, and it would be a difficult challenge to be able to describe them all. For environmental awareness of sound (e.g., phone calls, doorbell, door knock,

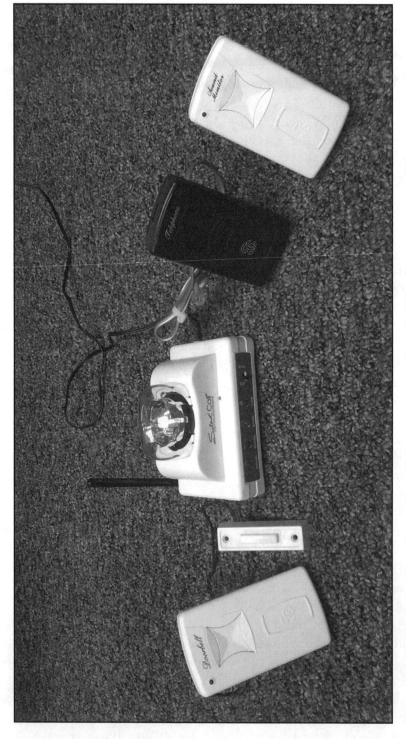

Figure 12–3. Example transmitter with multiple receivers by Silent Call Communications, Inc. The transmitter has a photo-electric strobe light station mounted on top. The receivers from left to right are doorbell signaler, telephone signaler, and sound monitor. Photo credit: Samuel R. Atcherson, PhD.

baby cry, etc.), individuals with hearing loss will need to consider if they need the sound made louder, or if an alternative flashing light or vibration signal would be better. Sometimes, both flashing lights and vibration modes are available in the same product. In some cases, these products are stand alone with built-in microphone signaling technology. In other cases, the microphone is part of a receiver, which then sends a signal to a transmitter containing the signaling technology (Figure 12–4). The same is true for motion detection signalers, which can be found in all-inclusive devices, or in a receiver/transmitter system. Potential customers should take time to explore options available from online distribution companies or other comparable retailers.

Mobile Phone Tip: Sound Monitor

There are some mobile apps designed to provide alerts for various environmental sounds. Apps Otosense, Hearing Aide, and MyEarDroid are all available in Google Play, while DeafAlarm is available in the Apple App Store. These apps may have algorithms to identify common household sounds, or for better accuracy, sounds may be recorded using the mobile phone and saved for future identification.

A clever product, called the Dream-Zon LightOn, is a tabletop device that has a cradle rest to place the mobile phone. For this product to work, the mobile phone must be set to vibrate mode, which allows the LightOn device to be sensitive only to the mobile phone's vibration

and not to other extraneous signals in the environment. Whenever there is an incoming SMS text, call, or video call, the LightOn device will detect the vibration and trigger a bright flashing light on the front and back of the device. The LightOn device can also work with an external transmitter that wirelessly transmits a signal to trigger a flashing light in another remote location in the home or office. For those who would like a vibration alert while sleeping, an external bed vibrator can also be connected to the LightOn.

Service Animals

"Is there an alternative to technology for alerting me to environmental sounds?"

A viable alternative to electronic alerting systems is the use of a service dog, a type of assistive dog (Figure 12–5). Service dogs for individuals with hearing loss (partner) are different from guide dogs, which are for individuals with vision impairments. Service dogs are specially trained to assist individuals with hearing loss by alerting them to specific environmental sounds. For example, service dogs will alert their partner to sounds commonly found in the home: fire and smoke alarms, telephone, oven timer, alarm clock, doorbell/door knock, and their name. They can also be trained to provide alerts for a baby cry, microwave, tea kettle, and washer/dryer. When out in public, service dogs can also alert their partners to other nonrepetitive sounds. For example, the partner may be alerted to other sounds by watching what his or her service dog may be reacting to.

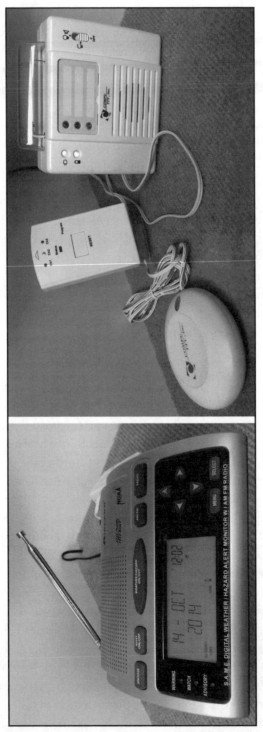

Figure 12–4. On the left is an example of a National Weather Radio (NWR) from Midland with an external weather alert transmitter (Krown KWA300TX) connected to the back. On the right is a Krown Wireless Alarm Monitoring KA300 system with KA300RX sound and strobe receiver and KBS300RX bed vibrator receiver. Both of these receivers will activate, for example, when the NWR and weather alert transmitter obtains alerts. Photo credit: Samuel R. Atcherson, PhD.

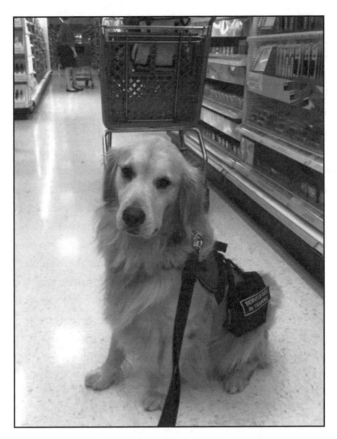

Figure 12–5. Example photo of a service dog in training at a grocery store. The vest indicates that the service dog is working and/or training. Image courtesy of http://www.pawsitivityservicedogs.com

There are a number of possible avenues available from agencies throughout the United States and other parts of the world to acquire a service dog. Interested individuals can first start their search by going to the Assistance Dog International website (http://www.assistancedogsinternational.org) and conducting a program search. While there may not be a program in each state, this website will list nearby programs. Each program varies slightly, but they all require completion of an application. Some may require a "good faith" refundable deposit after a fixed length of time in which the partner demonstrates that a good symbiotic relationship has formed and proper care of the dog was exhibited. The training of a service dog can take up to 18 months and may be customized. Certain breeds may be preferred.

Regardless of the type of service animal (vision, hearing, or other disability), it is important to know some basic etiquette. Service dogs are working dogs first, but they will be treated with many of the same freedoms as nonservice dogs. They will still enjoy treats, playtime and exercise, and being petted in appropriate situations. The bond between a service dog and partner will be a friendship for years to come. Service dogs have a special vest that allows them to be distinguished from nonservice dogs. This designation allows these service dogs access to locations such as restaurants and government buildings, which generally prohibit pets. When service dogs are working, they are not to be interacted with directly (i.e., offered food, water, or petted), at least not without the permission of the partner.

Summary

In this brief chapter, we reviewed a number of alerting devices and services. Whereas normal hearing listeners can depend on a wide variety of signals, individuals with hearing loss may require sound volume enhancement, try alternative light and vibration modalities, or adopt a service dog. Each of these devices and services aim to ensure that individuals with hearing loss have access to everyday sounds as well as emergency alerts. The capabilities of mobile phones are continually being tapped, not only for telecommunications, work, and entertainment, but also for promoting independence for individuals with hearing loss.

PART IV

Cases and Further Considerations

13

Case Studies

Introduction

In this chapter, we present in narrative format a variety of realistic cases of known and anticipated challenges, and possible solutions for them with respect to hearing loss. The cases below are examples in the schools, the workplace, as well as public and private settings. The cases also show how hearing assistive and access technologies can be used on both personal and public levels. The takeaway point is to see beyond the hearing aids and implantable devices to additional devices that may improve auditory (and sometimes visual) access, promote greater independence, and enhance quality of life. Readers are encouraged to spend time also with Chapter 5 on needs assessment as a supplement to this chapter.

The Schools

Case 1—Rebecca, Elementary School to Middle School

Rebecca is 11 years old and currently a sixth grader at a public school, Pinnacle Mountain Elementary School. She was diagnosed with a moderate to moderately severe hearing loss (pure tone average of ~56 dB HL) in both ears at age 3. Her hearing in both ears has changed over the years to what is now a severe hearing loss (~74 dB HL). Despite the severity of her hearing loss, she has had age-appropriate speech and language abilities and she relies quite heavily on lipreading to supplement what she hears. Rebecca wears behind-the-ear (BTE) hearing aids in both ears. Her hearing aids have three programs: (1) a "quiet" program for when there is little to no background noise, (2) a "noise" program using digital noise reduction and directional microphones for noisier environments, and (3) a "telephone" program that activates the hearing aid telecoil (t-coil) and deactivates the hearing aid microphone. These are typical features in many hearing aids that provide amplification of speech and environmental sounds, while attempting to improve signal-to-noise ratio (SNR) or provide listening comfort. Because of the severity of Rebecca's hearing loss, she greatly benefits from the built-in telecoil for telephone use and when using music headphones. When she activates the telecoil, she can focus completely on the telephone and on her music because the microphone is programmed to turn off. It also helps that the home telephone and her parent's mobile phones are all hearing aid compatible.

At Pinnacle Mountain Elementary School, Rebecca stays in one classroom with one teacher for most of her subjects, including English, History, Math, Science, and Language Arts. Occasionally, the class leaves for other activities such as Music and other school-wide events. In the classroom, desks are positioned in groups of four facing together, and with 32 students in the class, there are eight groups of tables spread throughout the classroom. Rebecca's Individualized Education Program (IEP) was established before the beginning of the school year by a team of her regular education teacher, an audiologist, and a speech-language pathologist, in consultation with her parents. Rebecca sits strategically in one of the grouped tables near the window and

the front of the classroom, but with her back facing the window. This seat arrangement does a few things. First, by having Rebecca's back face the window, it helps to avoid the teacher having a shadow cast on his face on bright, sunny days. Second, it maximizes audibility and visibility for listening to the teacher near the front of the room where the teacher will be spending most of his time. Finally, the seating position allows Rebecca to maximize visual access to other students in the room as opposed to having them all behind her if she were to sit in the front and center of the classroom. In addition to having occasional follow-up hearing, speech, and language evaluations, the IEP calls for continued use of a frequency-modulated (FM) (newer technology known as digital-modulated [DM]) system during all instruction times.

Rebecca previously used an FM system furnished by the school system's educational audiologist with an FM receiver that could be connected to her hearing aids while the teacher used a microphone transmitter. This FM system worked great because she could hear the teacher, Mr. Morse, at all times no matter where he was in the room. However, she could never take it for use outside of school. Recently, Rebecca and her parents learned from the educational audiologist, Dr. Jean, about hearing aids with an integrated (built-in) FM receiver and personal microphone transmitter that could be used both at school and outside of school. Rebecca and her family consulted with their primary audiologist to explore further. Rebecca was already due for new hearing aids, so it made sense to pursue a pair of hearing aids with integrated FM receivers and to get two different microphone transmitters: one for teachers at school and one for personal use. The microphone transmitter for the teacher had a belt or pocket model with a clip-on lapel microphone placed within 6 inches of the teacher's mouth. The personal microphone transmitter could be used in similar situations outside of the classroom. For example, during a school function involving a visit to a local art gallery, the tour guide would wear the microphone. The same personal microphone transmitter had some other interesting features that would allow Rebecca to hear on the phone wirelessly without holding the phone to her ear as well as use a portable music player or listen to computer sounds wirelessly. In other words, the information picked up by the personal microphone transmitter would be sent wirelessly to the hearing aids. Rebecca had an opportunity to try new hearing aids and the microphone transmitter options. In consultation with the audiologist, Rebecca had some new technology to look forward to, and one that would be hers to use both at school and at home.

In the classroom, Rebecca also benefited from other available access technologies such as closed captioning or subtitles on videos shown during class time. While this provides speech-to-text access, Rebecca also likes to have her teacher place the microphone transmitter next to the loudspeaker to give her auditory access as well.

Rebecca and her parents are now trying to prepare her for seventh grade at a nearby middle school. Until now, Rebec-

ca's parents woke her up every morning at 5:45 AM. Now, they want Rebecca to learn to become more independent in the comfort of their home. Prior to the start of the school year, Rebecca's parents will purchase a vibrating alarm clock and have her practice using it well in advance. Second, middle school involves multiple subjects taught by different teachers in different rooms. Rebecca will need to carry the microphone transmitter from class to class, increasing her responsibility to ensure that it stays charged and in good working order, and to report malfunctions to a designated person (e.g., IEP case manager, school audiologist, or school speech-language pathologist), and to her parents. Similar to the seating arrangement in elementary school, Rebecca needs to identify the best place to sit in each classroom so that she will be able to see both the teacher and the majority of other students in the classroom.

Although Rebecca and her parents are nervous about the transition from elementary to middle school, Rebecca feels prepared to handle these new responsibilities, ensure good auditory access and seating arrangements, and take advantage of the microphone transmitter options available to her for school and personal use. See Table 13–1.

Case 2—Anne, Nontraditional College Student Returning to School

Anne is a 31-year-old, returning nontraditional college student attempting to finish her bachelor's degree at Arkansas

Table 13–1. Case 1—Summary of Technology and Services

Technology and/or Service	Chapter	Description
Hearing aid	4	Hearing device that provides custom-fitted acoustic amplification with programmable channels for different listening needs
Telecoil	7	Permits use with hearing aid compatible phones and music headphones (also useful with induction hearing loops)
FM system	6	One of several wireless technologies to improve signal-to-noise ratio (SNR) using a microphone transmitter and a receiver (either coupled to the hearing device or built into the hearing device)
Closed captions/subtitles	11	Written text available during broadcast television programs, or preinstalled on visual media
Alarm clock signaler	12	Specially designed alarm clock systems designed to provide enhanced or novel stimuli (increased sound intensity, light, and/or vibrations) for deaf and hard of hearing consumers
Individualized education plan	2	Customized objectives for primary and secondary education students with disabilities, including hearing loss
Audiology	n/a	Personal and educational hearing-based intervention and management
Speech therapy	n/a	Personal and/or educational speech and language-based intervention and management

University. She has a profound sensorineural hearing loss, communicates orally, and wears a cochlear implant in each ear, which she received at separate times while in her late 20s. Although not her primary mode of communication, Anne has social command of sign language that she learned and used during her middle and high school years with school friends who were Deaf. In her primary and secondary school years, Anne wore hearing aids and was able to use a frequency-modulated (FM) system that connected directly to the back of her hearing aids using a small clip-on boot. She recalls hating having to wear this device, but she wore it diligently in her classes during formal instruction. She also recalls how difficult it was to engage in groups whether for in-class group assignments or out and around on campus, such as in the cafeteria. Anne feels fortunate that her friends made an effort to include her and keep her apprised of the topics of their discussion. Although a high-B student in high school, her first two years of college were unsuccessful at a small community college. She was also far from her family and friends, who were not able to offer their usual support. As a consequence she struggled to keep up with the pace and rigor of her classes, her grades began to suffer, and she dropped out of college.

What Anne did not realize, and was unprepared for, was a change in the treatment of individuals with disabilities by the schools. In her primary and secondary education years, the schools were responsible for her under the Individuals with Disabilities Education Act (IDEA), which addresses the educational needs of children with disabilities. The IDEA, in concert with Title II of the Americans with Disabilities Act (ADA), has a number of provisions: free and appropriate mandatory education, identification services, evaluations free to the student, development and implementation of an individualized education plan (IEP), advocacy provided by educators, and outcome-oriented learning. In postsecondary education, however, IDEA no longer applies, but certain provisions offered by the Rehabilitation Act of 1973 (Section 504) do apply, in addition to Title II. (See Chapter 2 for more information on these laws.) In contrast to the provisions offered by the IDEA for primary and secondary education school years, postsecondary education students are considered to have pursued optional education; they must self-disclose their disability in order to obtain services, they generally must provide some documentation of the disability, reasonable accommodations will be determined, students must self-advocate, and while there may be equal access,

there is no guarantee of equal outcomes. Thus, Anne and her family had not been prepared for the transition from high school to college. Nevertheless, Anne's confidence and communication abilities improved enough with her cochlear implants that she decided to go back and finish her college degree. A little older, and a little wiser, Anne began exploring options to maximize her success in college.

After spending some time exploring the different postsecondary institutions in her state, she was pleased to learn about a very knowledgeable and capable Disability Resource Center at Arkansas University. Compared to what happened almost a decade ago, Anne made the first contact by disclosing her disability and providing documentation. Prior to enrolling in classes, Anne and a Disability Resource Center staff member, Mr. Allen, discussed various accommodations that might be useful to her. Anne provided a copy of her audiogram, including hearing test information on her performance with cochlear implants. Even with cochlear implants, Anne admitted that she struggles with some people and the way they speak, and worries that she might not understand some professors as well as she would like. She recalled her days of using an FM system in high school, but even then she had great difficulty keeping up with her teachers because she would miss information any time she started taking notes. Mr. Allen recommended continuing to use an FM system to improve the signal-to-noise ratio in the classroom, but worried that some professors might not comply with the use of a microphone transmitter. Anne indicated that her cochlear implants had telecoils, and Mr. Allen said that they had induction neckloops and stock FM systems to loan to students each semester. Mr. Allen explained that the FM system may be useful in other situations outside of the classroom, such as university-wide sponsored lectures and while studying with friends. As a general rule, Mr. Allen also encouraged Anne to consult with her audiologist for other hearing augmentation options that he may not have considered.

Because of the note-taking issue, the Disability Resource Center staff member also recommended speech-to-text services, something Anne had never heard of. Mr. Allen said that two Disability Resource Center staff members were trained to provide speech-to-text services in the classroom. He explained how this worked: The student props a wireless tablet device with a preinstalled app on his or her desk. In the classroom, the speech-to-text provider will have set up a laptop to use somewhere in the classroom in a location that is not a distraction to the students and does not obstruct the activities of the class. After the class is over, the speech-to-text provider breaks down the equipment and leaves for the next classroom, all without Anne's direct involvement. When the class is in session, the speech-to-text provider transcribes what is said during the session regardless of who is speaking. In real time, Anne would see nearly everything spoken during the class on the tablet device. To get the tablet device to receive the information, Anne would receive an Internet Protocol (IP) address (e.g., 192.168.10.1) to enter into

the app to establish communication with the speech-to-text provider's laptop. Anne would also have to ensure that her tablet was connected to the Wi-Fi on campus. From there, Mr. Allen further described some of the benefits of speech-to-text technology. First, Anne would now have equal access to things said in the classroom, not only through sound, but also with visual support. Second, the full transcription of the class period can be sent to her school e-mail address as notes. Third, whenever uncaptioned videos or audio samples are played during class, the speech-to-text technology would provide access to that as well. Mr. Allen, however, encouraged her to continue to take her own notes as best she could, but to be selective about her note taking for recall purposes when she studied with the full transcription at a later time. He also told her that if she had a smartphone, she could install the same app as a backup, but the screen size would be a lot smaller. Anne was excited about having access to both an FM system to use with her cochlear implant, and the speech-to-text technology.

Being unmarried, Anne also decided to pursue nontraditional, on-campus student housing so that she could focus solely on her education for the next two to three years. In conversations with Mr. Allen about getting back into school, she made mention of her desire to live on campus. Mr. Allen mentioned that University Housing had a few rooms outfitted with a doorbell light signaler and a strobe light assembly in the rooms connected to the building's fire alarm system. If she were interested in such a room, Anne was encouraged to discuss this with University Housing. The obvious benefit here would be to respond either to her door or to emergencies any time she had her cochlear implants off. Anne indicated that she would be using her bed vibrating alarm clock to help her get up in the morning. For important situations such as taking an early morning test, she would also double up by setting the vibrating alarm on her smart phone. Mr. Allen was pleased to learn that Anne was already aware of alarm clock options, but offered to share with her a newer alarm system that works with a vibration-capable mobile or smartphone. Here the alarm clock has a built-in audible ringer, flashing light, and optional bedshaker, and all Anne would have to do is place her mobile smartphone in its cradle. When the phone vibrates, the new alarm system produces an audible signal and/or begins flashing the strobe light. If the optional bedshaker is used, Anne would also be alerted through vibration in the same manner as her current vibrating alarm clock.

Mr. Allen asked Anne about how she plans to communicate with her professors and other students. Anne indicated that e-mail would be her first choice, and if available, she would use text messaging and online social media messages to communicate. Although she is comfortable using the phone with her relatives and close friends, she stated that she tends to avoid using the phone. However, her Deaf friends introduced her to videophone and video relay services and she has a device set up at home that allows her to communicate with her Deaf friends by videophone. She admitted, however, that she was not comfortable using video relay services. Since Anne appeared interested in the speech-to-text technology in the classroom, he introduced her to some newer desktop telephone options that would allow her to use her own voice and to hear the person on the phone while also receiving a transcription of what her conversation partner said. Before pursuing a desktop phone, Mr. Allen encouraged her to try out one or more of these apps on her smartphone with a strong Wi-Fi connection.

Anne had no idea about some of the technologies Mr. Allen described, but she wanted to be sure to try them all at least once. She was glad that her comparison of different colleges led her to learning about the Disability Resource Center at Arkansas University. Anne is now excited about the prospects of doing well in school as she works toward the completion of her college degree. See Table 13–2.

The Workplace

Each state's Vocational Rehabilitation (VR) office is one of the most important services for hearing health care professionals and individuals with hearing loss to obtain hearing solutions for the workplace. VR services are intended to help individuals not only obtain work but also to remain in a job. Hence, seeking VR services if one is already employed but is having difficulties related to hearing loss

Table 13–2. Case 2—Summary of Technology

Technology and/or Service	Chapter	Description
Cochlear implants	4	Hearing device that provides custom-fitted electrical stimulation with programmable channels for different listening needs
Telecoil	7	Permits use with hearing aid compatible phones and music headphones (also useful with induction hearing loops)
FM System	6	One of several wireless technologies to improve signal-to-noise ratio (SNR) using a microphone transmitter and a receiver (either coupled to the hearing device or built into the hearing device)
Induction neckloop	7	One of several wireless technologies to improve signal-to-noise ratio (SNR). The induction neck loop emits an electromagnetic signal that is picked up by the hearing device telecoil.
Speech-to-text captioning	11	Written text provided using a real-time captionist who is able to hear everything spoken in a room and who types the information for the student to read on a screen
Tablet or smartphone device	n/a	Although commonplace, a tablet or smart device can be an extension of access technology using Wi-Fi or other short-range communication
Speech-to-text telephone	11	Unique telephone using a service that allows an operator to transcribe into visual text what is said by the person with whom you are speaking on the telephone
Doorbell signaler	12	Signaler connected to the doorbell (or add on) that provides a recognizable visual input that someone is at the door
Fire alarm signaler	12	Signaler connected to the smoke/fire alarm system (or add on) that provides a recognizable visual input
Alarm clock signaler	12	Specially designed alarm clock systems designed to provide enhanced or novel stimuli (increased sound intensity, light, and/or vibrations) for deaf and hard of hearing consumers

is a viable alternative funding source for hearing assistive and access technologies. Audiologists should understand the rules, regulations, and referral opportunities for VR in their state, in case a client needs that referral. In addition to other types of patients and patient referrals, audiologists may see clients who are referred by VR. If

VR is used as the funding source, remember this caveat: because the purpose of VR is to help people with employment, VR cannot pay for devices for the home or recreational use. Also, VR in each state has a limited budget; whether VR can fund requests for assistance will depend on the budget and the severity of the disability for everyday function.

Audiologists can best help clients by identifying and creatively addressing all the situations in the workplace that are problematic for that client. These situations will likely change based on a person's hearing status, occupation and particular workplace; therefore, using the most specific information possible for each client will yield the best results for that person.

Case 3—Frank, Hard of Hearing Sales Manager

Frank is a 63-year-old sales manager for a wind turbine blade manufacturing company. Frank has a long-standing sensorineural mild sloping to moderate hearing loss bilaterally and has worn in-the-ear hearing aids for many years. His hearing aids, along with a volume control on his landline office phone, have been sufficient accommodations for work. Lately, he has noticed he is having more difficulty than in the past. When he sees his audiologist for a hearing evaluation, Frank relays the following information: He can still fairly easily converse with one to two people when he can watch their faces, but in larger groups, he discovered that he misses important parts of the conversation because he cannot identify the speaker quickly enough to speechread them. Because of this *new* limitation, informal meetings have become challenging, and Frank has begun to avoid these situations. Formal meetings are problematic mainly for the same reason: finding the person who is speaking is not easy, and sitting around the meeting table prevents Frank from speechreading some of the other attendees based on where they are sitting. Frank has begun using a mobile phone often in the course of the day. Talking on the mobile phone can be difficult depending on the speaker. Hearing the phone ring is also an issue; he keeps his mobile phone on both vibrate and ring modes to help overcome this issue. With his long-standing hearing loss, Frank does not try to hide his communication issues at work; however, the demand on him to function at the same level with no additional help is stressful and tiring, which has also impacted his home life.

The hearing evaluation reveals that Frank's pure tone high-frequency thresholds have worsened, and his hearing loss is now in the mild sloping to moderately severe range. His word recognition in quiet, at a comfortable level of 80 dB HL, is comparable to his last evaluation four years prior. However, his ability to understand speech in background noise, using the QuickSIN test, is poorer with a signal-to-noise ratio (SNR) loss of 12 dB on today's evaluation (versus a SNR loss of 5 dB four years ago), objectively confirming the increased difficulty Frank has been experiencing. The audiologist reminds Frank to always use good communication strategies such as facing the speaker (to speechread), turning down or off background sounds when possible, and positioning himself advantageously for listening. This last recommendation will vary based on the setting Frank is in, and also the strengths of his communication partner(s). Educating the employees of Frank's company on communication strategies with a person who has hearing loss is also a possibility, although one that Frank is, understandably, not too keen on. However, an online employee program on working with individuals with a variety of disabilities may be helpful for them both inside and outside the company.

Frank has health insurance that will purchase two hearing aids up to $2,500 with a $500 co-pay, every four years. Because many of Frank's issues are work related, his audiologist explains the VR program and encourages Frank to submit an application. In addition, Frank's company will likely bear some of the cost for any needed assistive equipment, given their responsibility to their employees under the Americans with Disabilities Act (ADA), which Frank's audiologist also explains.

As a first step in the treatment plan, Frank's audiologist recommends small, behind-the-ear, thin-tube hearing aids. When Frank tries these on in the audiologist's office, he is surprised by the immediate increased clarity of the audiologist's speech, even in the relative quiet of the office. These hearing aids operate together to determine the best gain and microphone configuration but can be set with user-determined programs for patient-specific needs.

Frank discusses with his audiologist how important mobile phone use is in his job. The audiologist tells Frank about Bluetooth connectivity that is available for these hearing aids. Depending on the application and manufacturer, the Bluetooth signal may be sent from a transmitter (e.g., mobile phone, computer, tablet, etc.) directly to the hearing aids or may be sent to an intermediate device typically worn around the neck or in a pocket, called a streamer. The mobile phone or other Bluetooth-enabled device sends the signal to the streamer, which then transfers the sound via either frequency-modulated (FM) or induction loop technology to the hearing aids. In addition to the mobile phone, and depending on the company, Bluetooth gives access to other devices such as portable music players, computers, radio, landlines, and television (although television use would require Frank to purchase the additional instrumentation needed for this application).

The audiologist explains that this particular model of hearing aid uses a 2.4 GHz wireless technology that works with an app designed for the iPhone, which is the brand of mobile phone Frank uses. This app will allow Frank to use the phone to adjust the volume of his hearing aids and also the treble and bass settings, to some extent. The app also allows for location-specific settings. For example, when Frank is at his favorite coffee shop, he can adjust the settings, save the location, and whenever he returns to that location the system returns the aids to Frank's preferred settings. The number of locations that the app will store is limited to two or three, however. The app lets the mobile phone function as a remote microphone, turning the mobile phone/hearing aid combination into an assistive device. In meetings with only a few people, Frank could place his mobile phone in the center of the table to capture the speakers' voices to be sent wirelessly to his hearing aids. The sensitivity of the mobile phone microphone will be the limiting factor in this setup. Another good feature of this app is a "find my hearing aid" capability. If Frank accidentally left his hearing aids somewhere, the app will list the last location that the aids were paired with the iPhone, for example, the office of the last client Frank met with. If he were to misplace his hearing aids within his home or office, the mobile phone app will send out a signal, allowing him to locate his hearing aids.

The in-house sales meetings Frank attends always occur in the same conference room. About 15 to 20 people generally attend this meeting, so the mobile phone as his remote microphone would be insufficient. Frank's company could "loop" this room, that is, install induction loop technology around the perimeter, allowing Frank to sit anywhere in the room and still have access to the signal through the telecoil in his aid, so long as the microphone(s) in use are tied to the induction system. This is not a problem for the main microphone located on the lectern but does present challenges if someone other than the person at the lectern is speaking. There are a couple of options in this case: First, the meeting etiquette could change such that whoever

wants to speak must go to the lectern. That solution is probably impractical, given the number of individuals in the meeting, but it may work. Second, it may be possible to install several microphones in various locations around the room and connect them to the room's sound system. Such a setup is likely to cover anyone speaking from any point in the room. The audiologist can certainly suggest this induction loop option to Frank, although it is unlikely the audiologist can set this up. Frank's company would do well to contact a local supplier of induction loop technology and work with their experts on the best solution for that particular room.

Other options for hearing assistive technology in that meeting room would be an infrared (IR) or FM system. The advantage of each of these systems would be that there are ear-level receivers available for individuals who do not wear hearing aids, or for individuals with hearing aids that do not have a telecoil. For Frank, these two systems may present a challenge, unless his hearing aids are equipped with an FM receiver and no hearing aids have infrared receivers. See Table 13–3.

Case 4—Sandy, Late Deafened, in a Retail Environment

Sandy is a 36-year-old mother of two with a congenital heart valve defect. She needed a root canal and was given, prophylactically, amikacin, an aminoglycoside antibiotic. Unknown to Sandy or her

Table 13–3. Case 3—Summary of Technology and/or Services

Technology and/or Service	Chapter	Description
Hearing aid	4	Hearing device that provides custom-fitted amplified acoustic stimulation with programmable channels for different listening needs
Telecoil	7	Permits use with hearing aid compatible phones and music headphones (also useful with induction hearing loops)
FM system	6	One of several wireless technologies to improve signal-to-noise ratio (SNR) using a microphone transmitter and a receiver (either coupled to the hearing device or built into the hearing device)
Induction neckloop	6	One of several wireless technologies to improve signal-to-noise ratio (SNR). The induction neck loop emits an electromagnetic signal that is picked up by the hearing device telecoil.
Smartphone device (app to control hearing aids)	n/a	Although commonplace, a tablet or smart device can be an extension of access technology using Wi-Fi or other short-range communication
Vocational rehabilitation services	n/a	Located in various departments by state, this office is charged with provision of counseling, training, education, transportation, job placement, assistive technology, and other support services for individuals with disabilities.

dentist, she has a genetic change in her mitochondrial DNA (1555A>G), giving her a predisposition to aminoglycoside ototoxicity. Within four days of taking the amikacin, Sandy lost hearing in both ears, leaving her with severe-to-profound sensorineural hearing loss, bilaterally. Sandy entered the hearing health care system at this point and opted to receive bilateral cochlear implants.

With her sudden, almost complete loss of hearing, Sandy has had difficulty adjusting to this new reality and feared for her future earning potential. She has worked as a salesperson in a high-end furniture establishment for 13 years and does not think she can continue in that line of work. Sandy is currently on unpaid leave through the Family and Medical Leave Act (FMLA) and her company is willing to work with Sandy. Recognizing that Sandy has needs beyond audiologic and communication help, her audiologist refers her to VR. From VR, Sandy receives referrals for a mental health assessment and regular sessions with a rehabilitation counselor for hard of hearing/late deafened consumers. The rehabilitation counselor can help Sandy adjust to the use of cochlear implants and other hearing assistive and access technologies, provide a job site and accommodations analysis, and, working with Sandy's audiologist, provide an assistive device assessment. Sandy's audiologist refers her to a support group for new cochlear implant users, the Hearing Loss Association of America (HLAA), which has a local chapter, and signs Sandy up for speechreading classes in his office.

Cochlear implants and hearing aids have the same accessibility options: FM receiver, telecoil, and wireless reception. Cochlear implants have an additional capability that may or may not exist with hearing aids: direct audio input—that is, a wire from an input device plugs into the processor. Depending on the manufacturer or model of the cochlear implant, the telecoil may be integrated into the circuitry of the cochlear implant and may or may not reside in one of the program settings. If the telecoil is outside the program settings, the user can engage the telecoil along with each program, giving the user more flexibility for receiving input through induction and into the microphone, FM receiver, or directly via wire. Most cochlear implants have a "standard" port for an FM receiver, often the same receiver that is used with hearing aids. There are several types of cables for direct audio input. For example, MED-EL has one cable that allows input from the cochlear implant microphone, to remain aware of environmental sounds, and a connected audio device, while a second cable provides input primarily (90%)

from the connected audio device with minimal microphone input (10%). Last, MED-EL offers a direct audio input cable that will attach to two cochlear implants, giving stereo sound from the connected audio device.

Sandy's loss of hearing is frightening to her, since she does not have any life experience with hearing loss. Rehabilitation counseling, support group interaction, and speechreading classes will be necessary to help her navigate this new world. In addition, because her company is willing to work with Sandy, employee instruction on interacting with someone with hearing loss may prove invaluable for Sandy's return to work. Whether she is able to continue as a salesperson may not be answerable until her return. Sandy will need to be proactive about her hearing loss with customers, at the very least ensuring good communication strategies, if not explaining her hearing loss and asking for particular communication techniques from the customers. Should that not work out, Sandy may be able to transfer to a different job function within this company. See Table 13–4.

Public and Private Settings

Case 5—Jennifer, Family Travel Adventure (Adult)

Jennifer, a 40-year-old wife and mother, has a mild-to-moderate sensorineural hearing loss with the greatest degree of

Table 13–4. Case 4—Summary of Technology and/or Services

Technology and/or Services	Chapter	Description
Cochlear implants	4	Hearing device that provides custom-fitted electrical stimulation with programmable channels for different listening needs
Telecoil	7	Permits use with hearing aid compatible phones and music headphones (also useful with induction hearing loops)
FM system	6	One of several wireless technologies to improve signal-to-noise ratio (SNR) using a microphone transmitter and a receiver (either coupled to the hearing device or built into the hearing device)
Induction neckloop	7	One of several wireless technologies to improve signal-to-noise ratio (SNR). The induction neckloop emits an electromagnetic signal that is picked up by the hearing device telecoil.
Direct audio input	n/a	Method to improve the signal-to-noise ratio (SNR) through direct hardwired transmission from an audio device to a receiver, such as a cochlear implant or other assistive device (e.g., PockeTalker)
Speechreading classes	n/a	Opportunity to learn how to use visual speech cues (visemes) with auditory information to improve access to spoken language

loss around 3000 Hz. She has worn hearing aids for most of her life; but, with some progression in her hearing loss, mostly in the high frequencies, Jennifer has found success with her new receiver-in-the-canal (RIC) hearing aids. She is especially thrilled with the different directional microphone settings and wireless capabilities of the hearing aids.

Today, Jennifer is traveling to a national park and a theme park with her family for an overdue vacation. With her hearing loss, she knows how difficult traveling can be, so she investigates and plans before the trip. She finds both her audiologist and the Internet to be valuable resources in planning the trip. During the initial part of the trip, Jennifer and her family must drive about an hour to catch a flight at a nearby airport. She knows how difficult it will be to hear the others while riding in the car with her husband driving and 6-year-old daughter in the back seat. Using her hearing aids' directional microphones and noise reduction technologies, Jennifer can better share in her family's excitement as they discuss the plans for their vacation.

Upon reaching the airport, Jennifer anticipates the visual paging system via digital video information boards and the assistive listening devices at the public airport, which comply with the Americans with Disabilities Act (ADA). From her previous experiences flying, she knows that this particular airport also has an increased number of public address loudspeakers. The increased number of loudspeakers, spread throughout the airport means that each loudspeaker is set at a slightly lower intensity level. This allows Jennifer and other hearing aid and implant device users to be closer to loudspeakers throughout the airport than if there were only a few centralized speakers. She knows this speaker arrangement makes it easier and more comfortable to hear, as airports can be quite loud. Because of her hearing loss, she requests preboarding privileges so that (1) she will not miss the boarding call, (2) she and her family can have the opportunity to locate their seats, and (3) speak with the airline flight crew before the other passengers come aboard and make noise. Again, Jennifer uses her hearing aids' directional microphones and noise reduction technologies to better communicate with her husband and daughter. Jennifer's flight connects with the second leg of her trip at a much larger airport. Jennifer was prepared for the potential communication challenges at this airport as she had been in the smaller airport. Prior to her trip, Jennifer investigated the methods this airport employs to assist those with hearing loss. She discovered that this airport uses an induction hearing loop system. She can use the telecoil (t-coil) in her hearing aids to directly pick up transmitted public address announcements, with very little interference. She knows that hearing boarding and other announcements will supplement the visual information regarding flight arrivals and takeoffs on the digital video information boards. As a conscientious mother and savvy traveler, she was relieved to discover that if an emergency were to occur during her time at this airport, these video boards would post important large bold messages about the emergency.

Leaving the airport via taxi to visit a national park, Jennifer appreciates that the taxicab has been modified with an induction hearing loop so that she can easily hear the driver, using the telecoil in her hearing aids. As the taxicab approaches the entrance to the park, Jennifer and her family contact the park's visitor information center to investigate the availability of assistive devices. The park provides Jennifer with an assistive listening device, which amplifies the nearby sounds in the environment and the prescripted narration with historical and park information at different locations throughout the park. While she has some issues using the stereo headphones that come with the device along with her hearing aids, Jennifer is still pleased with what she can hear. In fact, she is amazed by the device's ability to provide the appropriate narration at the most opportune times throughout the park. The device uses different forms of wireless communications, including a Global Positioning System (GPS), allowing the facility to provide the appropriate narration at strategic locations around the park area.

The next day, Jennifer and her family head to a major theme park. Coincidentally, this park uses the same device as the one she used at the national park. This time, she discovers that the device will also work with an induction neckloop and the telecoil in her hearing aids. Jennifer is able to share in all of the experiences of the theme park, including the dizzying rides, with her family. At the end of the day, her entire family is drained, but happy, as they plan to head back home. Jennifer and her family have such a positive experience that they decide to vacation in the same location the following year. With all of the challenges of travel and family vacations, Jennifer was glad that she researched and utilized all of the hearing assistive and access technologies available for her trip. See Table 13–5.

Table 13–5. Case 5—Summary of Technology and/or Services

Technology and/or Services	Chapter	Description
Hearing aid	4	Hearing device that provides custom-fitted amplified acoustic stimulation with programmable channels for different listening needs
Visual paging system	n/a	Digital video information boards, usually providing takeoff and arrival times, can also be used to relay emergency information to those unable to hear announcements
Assistive listening devices	6–9	A variety of devices that are capable of receiving, amplifying, and transmitting/delivering a signal to facilitate listening
Cochlear implant	4	Hearing device that provides custom-fitted electrical stimulation with programmable channels for different listening needs
Induction loop system	7	One of several wireless technologies to improve signal-to-noise ratio (SNR). The induction neckloop emits an electromagnetic signal that is picked up by the hearing device telecoil.
Telecoil	7	Permits use with hearing aid compatible phones and music headphones (also useful with induction hearing loops)
Wireless communications	9	Any method for two devices to transmit and receive transmission other than with the use of wires (e.g., Bluetooth)

Case 6—Meghan, Family Travel Adventure (Child)

Meghan is a young girl with a moderate sensorineural hearing loss. She has worn behind-the-ear (BTE) hearing aids for a few years with reasonable success. Meghan heads to New York City with her parents for a long getaway weekend. They plan to enjoy the city's abundance of cultural experiences, including art, dining, sports, and shopping. The first part of their trip includes travel via train from her hometown to New York City. Meghan's parents let her know that she can use the telecoil (t-coil) function of her hearing aids to hear announcements both on the train and in the station, which have both been outfitted with induction hearing loop technology. While Meghan could care less about these announcements, she is excited that the train offers free Wi-Fi. Now, she can create an internet-of-things (IOT) using her tablet and hearing aids. Her tablet and hearing aids are connected via Bluetooth, so she can hear the audio from the tablet directly in her ears without having to hear the noise from the train. With a few hours on the train, Meghan had planned to watch a movie and some recent shows that she had missed on television. She had also thought about using Skype or FaceTime to catch up with her friends from school. An hour into the trip, Meghan's parents insist that she put down her tablet and spend some quality time with them. As she reluctantly agrees, she adjusts her hearing aids' program for noisy listening situations with directional microphones. Instantly, she realizes the improvement over her basic hearing aid program, which has settings appropriate for quiet listening environments.

Meghan and her family arrive in New York City and head straight for Yankee Stadium for a baseball showdown between the New York Yankees and the Boston Red Sox. Because Yankee Stadium provides listening assistance via induction loop technology, Meghan does not miss any of the action. She and her dad keep score and discuss batting order as they all enjoy America's favorite pastime. After the game, they decide to enjoy one of the city's fine dining experiences. Similar to listening on the train, the noise presents a problem. This time, Meghan's hearing aids are not enough to overcome the noise from others in the restaurant talking. Meghan's mom suggests that she use her remote microphone. At first, Meghan's parents pass the microphone back and forth, taking turns to speak. After the food arrives at the table, they decide to use the remote microphone only as needed. At this point in the meal, no one is talking much as they eat.

The next day, Meghan and her family wake early, using a portable vibrating alarm that, when placed under the pillow, wakes her with a vibrating shake. Today's primary destination includes a trip to the Guggenheim Museum. They stop at the Media Guide desk for assistance and discover that induction loop technology provides narration for information about the exhibits and even architecture. Using her hearing aids' telecoil, Meghan can learn and enjoy throughout the museum. There is even assistance in the Peter B. Lewis

Theatre, which uses an infrared (IR) system and a neckloop that works with the telecoil in Meghan's hearing aids. A day of art is followed by an evening of basketball at the Barclays Center Arena. Again, Meghan is able to maximize her experience and enjoy her time with her parents as the center also provides induction loop technology. With all of the excitement from a busy day, Meghan found that she was most excited to be able to hear the concessions vendor when ordering a hot dog and soda. They used a countertop induction loop system. While waiting in the concession vendor line, she is still able to capture the highlights of the game on a nearby television screen with live closed captioning. On the third day of her long weekend, Meghan and her family visit the botanical gardens. While the gardens offer induction loop technology, Meghan and her parents decide to use the remote microphone. Unlike the noise in the restaurant, the gardens are serene, and after the excitement of the past couple of days, Meghan and her family decide to limit their discussions and enjoy nature's beauty. The trip to the big city was exciting, but not overwhelming, thanks to all of the hearing assistive and access technology provided for this young girl and other customers with hearing loss. See Table 13–6.

Table 13–6. Case 6—Summary of Technology and/or Services

Technology and/or Service	Chapter	Description
Hearing aid	4	Hearing device that provides custom-fitted amplified acoustic stimulation with programmable channels for different listening needs
Remote microphone	4, 9	A hearing aid accessory (i.e., microphone) placed near the sound source, resulting in less interference
Assistive listening devices	6–9	A variety of devices that are capable of receiving, amplifying, and transmitting/delivering a signal to facilitate listening
Telecoil	7	Permits use with hearing aid compatible phones and music headphones (also useful with induction hearing loops)
Hearing loop technology	7	One of several wireless technologies to improve signal-to-noise ratio (SNR) The induction neckloop emits an electromagnetic signal that is picked up by the hearing device telecoil.
Infrared system	8	Devices that transmit a signal via light waves
Wireless communications	9	Method for two devices to transmit and receive signals without the use of wires (e.g., Bluetooth, Wi-Fi, etc.)

Case 7—Tony and Leigh, Newlyweds and Communication

Tony, a man in his mid-20s, has recently married. He has a mild, sloping to moderate sensorineural hearing loss due mostly to noise exposure, as he is an avid wood-worker and hunter and he fails to use hearing protection during his hobbies. Not long ago, he mentioned to his audiologist that he learned the value of his hearing and the importance of protecting his residual hearing. He has worn in-the-ear hearing aids with some success; however, one of Tony's biggest challenges involves watching television and entertaining in his den. The room is long and narrow with the television on the wall farthest from his sofa. He researched and purchased a television appropriate for this distance. His current complaint is that although he can see the television, he has trouble hearing it, especially when others are talking in the room. He also has difficulty understanding friends and his wife, Leigh, when socializing in the den. He now avoids the room that he thought would be his favorite of the whole house.

In the den, there are large windows on one wall. He likes the light and openness from the windows, as it makes the room appear larger. The windows have no window treatments, such as blinds, valances, or curtains. The other walls in the room are essentially bare, except for a poster of his favorite football team. The floor is bare, except for a small doormat. Tony discusses his situation with his audiologist. For this particular appointment, he brings his wife to accompany him.

Between the couple and the audiologist, they realize that the room is highly reverberant, meaning that the sound in the room reflects from all of the bare surfaces. In most home listening environments, some reverberation provides richness and sound quality. While the reverberation in this room makes music sound nice, when people speak, there is a hollow and unnatural quality. The reverberation in this room makes it difficult to understand what other people in the room are saying. Leigh uses this information, along with some decorating ideas, to modify the décor of the room. First, she adds some area rugs to the floor, and with help from Tony, she installs window treatments on the windows. Then, they buy a couple of paintings and a tapestry for the other walls in the room. While this art is visually pleasant, it also is made of sound absorbing material such as cloth/fabric. The room is much more pleasant for everyone, especially Tony.

Although hearing and listening in the den have improved, Tony decides to purchase a wireless accessory for his hearing aids specifically designed to improve listening to the television, as well as a remote microphone for listening to others. These devices work with his hearing aids via wireless communication. Tony now experiences more comfortable listening and better understanding when he relaxes in the den.

Recently, Tony and Leigh suffer from a common communication challenge for married couples. They tend to speak/shout to one another when in different rooms, which removes powerful visual communication cues. Although Tony's audiologist counseled the couple about good communication strategies, the couple cannot break the bad habit of communicating with each other from different rooms. Leigh, being tech savvy, decided to purchase some Bluetooth-enabled light bulbs/speakers. With a smart device app, she can speak to Tony from any other room in the house. Her efforts were noble, but not successful, as there was some time delay in the signal and Tony would still have to shout back to her. Nevertheless, they kept the light bulb/speakers because they liked the technology. During a follow-up visit to the audiologist, Tony learns of an interesting mobile phone app. It will even deliver the signal directly to his hearing aids. He and Leigh can use the app to make their smartphones or tablets into walkie-talkies. Now, when Leigh is at the other end of the house and wants to talk with Tony, she speaks to him via the app. This works great if they have prepared to use the app. They have now agreed to have at least one device with each of them when Tony watches television and Leigh is in another room, or vice versa. This has taken some effort, and is far from perfect communication, but for brief interactions, the smart device app has made communication from different parts of the house better for the young couple. See Table 13–7.

Summary

The seven case studies presented in this chapter cover a number of different scenarios where various hearing assistive and access technologies are used. In each case, scenarios were described involving technologies (and services) well beyond hearing aids and implantable devices. Each scenario is reflective of technologies available today, all of which have been addressed in this book. We remind readers to view each individual with hearing loss uniquely, but holistically by conducting a needs assessment (see Chapter 5). We are excited about what the future holds with newer, cutting-edge communication technologies. Chapter 15

Table 13–7. Case 7—Summary of Technology and/or Services

Technology and/or Service	Chapter	Description
Hearing aid	4	Hearing device that provides custom-fitted amplified acoustic stimulation with programmable channels for different listening needs
Remote microphone	4, 9	A hearing aid accessory (i.e., microphone) placed near the sound source, resulting in less interference
Wireless communications	9	Any method for two devices to transmit and receive transmission other than with the use of wires (e.g., Bluetooth)

showcases some of the cutting-edge technology that is available today.

We believe that every person has a right to communication access for educational, vocational, and social purposes. These technologies have the power to decrease dependence, enhance quality of life, encourage and maintain a social life, and even prevent cognitive declines associated with hearing loss. It will take hearing and related professionals, as well as individuals with hearing loss and their communities, to increase awareness of these technologies and continually advocate for equal access, even if equal outcomes cannot be achieved.

14

Health Professionals With Hearing Loss

Overview

With inspiration from the Association of Medical Professionals with Hearing Losses (AMPHL) and the Association of Audiologists with Hearing Loss (AAHL), this chapter focuses strictly on health professionals with hearing loss. The health care industry is one of the fastest growing, and the demands placed on health professionals are high. The ability to communicate and share accurate information with the patient, families, and other health professionals is paramount. Depending on job expectations, health professionals may also need to rely on specialized hearing assistive and access technology to perform their job tasks.

There is ample evidence that the number of health professionals and stu-

dents with hearing loss is increasing (Dietrich, 2005; Larkin, 2009; Moreland, Latimore, Sen, Arato, & Zazove, 2013; Rhodes, Davis, & Odom, 1999; Velde, Chapin, & Wittman, 2005; Yoder & Pratt, 2005). This is due in part to advances in education, communication access, and assistive listening device and alerting systems. The increase is also due in part to legal or civil protections and opportunities for persons with disabilities who are otherwise able and/or qualified to train and practice (e.g., *Argenyi v. Creighton University*, 2013). The health professional or student with hearing loss may require a nonconventional stethoscope, alternative options to face masks that do not obscure the mouth and lips, and different communication and telecommunication solutions compared to health professionals who do not have hearing loss. In this chapter, we cover special considerations and technologies for health professionals with hearing loss. In addition, we offer a special spotlight on audiologists with hearing loss as it relates to their work involving sound and communication disorders.

Although there may be parallels for workers in other vocations (readers are directed to Morris, 2007), the special focus of this chapter on health professionals with hearing loss is due to the broad diversity of and roles for various health professionals focused on the care of human or animal patients. Health professionals must interact with patients, their families, and other health professionals. They work in a wide variety of settings from small, private examination rooms to large, open emergency areas. Depending on the setting, the equipment used, and the physical layout of the facility, background noise may be a significant problem. As a side note, recent studies suggest that hospitals are noisier places than they were 50 years ago, which can reportedly affect health workers' stress levels and patient rest and recovery (Busch-Vishniac et al., 2005; Falk & Woods, 1973). With respect to hearing loss, background noise can also affect communication and the ability to detect important signals and code alerts, which only compounds the challenge.

Needs of Health Professionals With Hearing Loss

Health professionals with hearing loss are not unlike any other patient or client with hearing loss. They all have various communication and access needs, and they can (and will) benefit from technologies and strategies that keep them employable and help them enjoy a reasonable quality of life. Health professionals with hearing loss will be a diverse group. There are health professionals who lose hearing long after they have completed their professional training and are already in the workforce. For these workers, the concern is shifted to trying to maintain clinical skills and competencies, and continue to advance in their fields. On the other hand, there are aspiring health professionals who experience hearing loss prior to or during their professional training. For students, there will often be a great deal of anxiety in the development of clinical knowledge, skills, and competencies. From an academic and training standpoint, the faculty and clinical instructors will be anticipating and periodically evaluating how the technical standards (also called essential functions) will be met and maintained. Technical standards should not be used in a manner that denies admission or continuation in the program simply on the basis of a disability. Rather, the student and program faculty should take steps to determine how those technical standards can be met with existing resources and technology in the form of reasonable accommodations. Although the goal is equal access to classroom and clinical training instruction, equal outcomes among students cannot be guaranteed. Whether in the vocational or training stage, communication and interprofessional relationships will remain important whether one's hearing loss remains unchanged or worsens over time.

For health professionals with hearing loss, having access to work-related sounds is an issue, but one that has a variety of solutions. At the most basic level, having the right personal amplification or implant device is the first step, whether becoming a first-time user or having a change or update in hearing technology. For those with severe to profound hearing losses whose primary communication modality is sign language, a hearing aid or cochlear implant may have limited use for spoken language communication, but instead would be used to provide access to work-related sounds such as auscultation and patient/safety alerting systems. When hearing aids and implantable devices are limited because of poor signal-to-noise ratio (SNR) issues (see Chapters 3 and 4), the health professional may be able to take advantage of other forms of auditory and/ or visual technologies, such as described in many of the chapters in this book. In order to avoid redundancy with other chapters, we focus here on stethoscopes, protective face masks, alerting systems, and designated interpreters as related to health professionals with hearing loss.

Stethoscopes

For such a small market, there are an impressive number of nonconventional stethoscopes available to health professionals with hearing loss. Stethoscopes are used to perform auscultation, which means to examine various body sounds acoustically, including the heart, lungs, bowels, arteries, and veins. Some may argue that stethoscopes will be a thing of past as the auscultation skills of physicians, nurses, and other allied health professionals decline with the rise of computer-assisted methods (e.g., echo-cardiography). Some skills, such as sphygmomanometry (blood pressure measurement), remain as common occurrences in physician offices and health clinics (Perloff et al., 1993). Proponents of auscultation skills cite that only through skilled listening can certain body sounds be judged to be benign or pathologic, and that well-performed auscultation keeps overall health costs down (Clark, Ahmed, Dell'Italia, Fan, & McGiffin, 2012). One can also not be at the mercy of electricity and other conveniences of modern-day technology. Thus, it is no surprise that fundamental auscultation skills continue to be taught in health care programs around the world.

Body sounds vary drastically in terms of intensity, frequency, and timbre (quality). For example, heart sounds are typically very low in frequency, between 5 and 200 Hz, whereas lung sounds are higher through about 2000 Hz. What many do not realize is that while human hearing sensitivity can range from 20 to 20,000 Hz in young, healthy individuals, we are most sensitive to speech sounds in the range of 100 to 8000 Hz. That is, we are much more sensitive to speech frequencies than we are the frequencies below and above the speech frequency range. Related to this point is that at very low and very high frequencies it takes more acoustic energy before these sounds become audible to the human ear. For example, at 1000 Hz it only takes about 10 dB SPL to detect the sound. Whereas at 50 Hz, the sound must be 50 to 60 dB SPL before one can detect the sound. As a general guide, the frequency ranges for various auscultation sounds are as follows: cardiovascular, 20 to 1000 Hz; pulmonary, 150 to 1000 Hz; gastrointestinal, 100 to 1000 Hz; and cervical, 75 to 1200 Hz.

To hear sounds from the surface of the body (e.g., chest wall, abdomen, or neck), a conventional acoustic stethoscope can help. However, extra fat or muscle, as well as background noise in the environment, can reduce the overall intensity, even for normal hearing listeners. It is for this reason that some clever advances have been made with stethoscopes by adding electronic amplifiers and/or noise reduction circuits. These electronic stethoscopes make it easier for both normal hearing listeners and some listeners with hearing loss. In some cases, listeners with hearing loss may be able to take their own hearing aids out and perform auscultation with an amplified stethoscope. For many, however, this is not always a desirable solution due to lack of convenience and the need to minimize the spread of infection. The inconvenience comes from having to take the hearing aids out, using the stethoscope, and then putting the hearing aids back in. For some, this creates a communication barrier between the health professional and the patient. Borrowing from a trick that some health professionals use with patients who have no more than a moderate hearing loss, it may be possible to use the conventional stethoscope as a temporary hearing aid. For example, the health professional will place the stethoscope ear tips into their patients' ears and then talk to them through the bell and diaphragm. This very act promotes understanding, which could increase consent and compliance. Likewise, the health professional with hearing loss could use the stethoscope in this way so as not to lose communicative contact with the patient during auscultation. Spread of infection could occur through poor infection control practices between physical contact with the patient during auscultation and handling one's hearing aids. To avoid removing one's hearing aids (or implant device) one or more alternative solutions may be available, but there is no one-size-fits-all approach. Table 14–1 lists some alternative approaches to consider involving the stethoscope ear tips, stethoscope ear tubes, or amplified stethoscope. For those interested in an amplified stethoscope, Table 14–2 lists a number of products currently on the market or being sold second-hand.

Potential consumers (and readers) should have a basic understanding of the decibel (dB) and amplification claims made by stethoscope manufacturers. Decibels are logarithmic numbers based on a reference point that represents the softest physical sound pressure that can be detected by normal hearing individuals. Any amount above that reference point is a ratio that reflects a change in loudness, sound pressure, or power, each of which yields very different values from a mathematical standpoint. Audio products are often reported in sound pressure level (SPL), not loudness or power. For example, if a manufacturer reports that their amplified stethoscope is "50 times louder" than a conventional,

Table 14–1. Alternative Uses of Stethoscopes With Hearing Aids and Implantable Devices

Approach	Descriptions
Stethoscope ear tips with conventional or amplified stethoscope	• Standard stethoscope ear tips may be placed directly into the ear canal while using open-ear, receiver-in-the canal, or deep-fitted completely-in-the canal (CIC) hearing aids.
	• A custom, behind-the-ear hearing aid earmold with negative impression divot (e.g., Westone Stethocut) could be used. See Figure 14–1.
Stethoscope ear tubes (ear tips removed) with conventional or amplified stethoscope	• With ear tips removed, a custom behind-the-ear hearing aid earmold could be made to accept the metal ends of the ear tubes.
	• With ear tips removed, a Westone Stetho-O-Mate could be substituted for use with deep-fitted completely-in-the-canal (CIC) hearing aids.
Audio output with amplified stethoscope	• Some amplified stethoscopes have an audio output jack to use a direct-audio input (DAI) patch cable, induction neckloop/silhouette, or headphones depending on the capabilities of the hearing aid (or implant device) and related accessories. For example, headphones may be placed directly over the hearing aid microphone to use acoustically, or the hearing aid telecoil may be activated to use an induction neckloop or headphone. Caution is advised when using telecoils as they have a low-frequency rolloff (see Chapter 7).

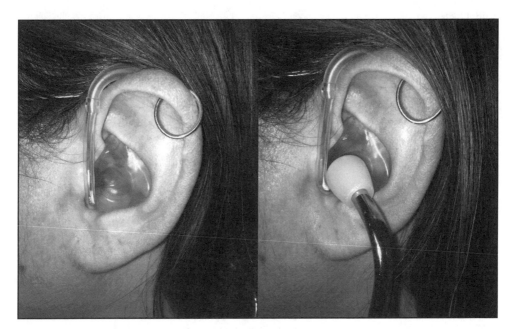

Figure 14–1. Behind-the-ear hearing aid with full-shell earmold customized with the Westone Stethocut to accept the ear tips of a listening scope or stethoscope. Photo credit: Kristen Kramer, AuD, CCC-A.

Table 14–2. Makes, Models, and Descriptions and Unique Features of Amplified and/or Visual Stethoscopes

Make and Model	Amplified or Visual	Description and Unique Features
American Diagnostic Corporation Adscope 657	Amplified	• Standard ear tips for conventional use • Sound output port for recording/ playback and attaching headphones for a second listener • <16× amplification
Cardionics E-scope Electronic Scope (Hearing-Impaired Model #718-7700)	Amplified	• Standard ear tips for conventional use • Sound output port for recording/playback and attaching headphones for a second listener • <30× amplification with maximum output of 125 dB
Cardionics E-scope Electronic Scope (Hearing-Impaired Model #718-7710)	Amplified	• Belt model; no standard ear tips • Sound output port for recording/playback and attaching headphones or patch cable (3.5 mm mono) • <30× amplification with maximum output of 125 dB
Cardionics E-scope EMS (Hearing-Impaired Model #718-7800)	Amplified	• Aviation-style (circumaural) headphones to minimize outside noise • <30× amplification with maximum output of 122 dB
Cardionics Vi-scope Electronic Scope (Hearing-Impaired Model #718-7910)	Both	• Phonocardiogram or phonopneumogram visual display • Standard ear tips for conventional use • <30× amplification
Littmann Electronic Stethoscope Model 3100 RM-LS3100	Amplified	• Ambient noise reduction • Frictional noise reduction • 24× amplification
Littmann Electronic Stethoscope Model 3200 with Bluetooth RM-LS3200	Both	• Ambient noise reduction • Frictional noise reduction • Bluetooth for wireless hearing and lung visualization • <24× amplification
ThinkLabs One	Amplified	• Multiple filter choices (digital selection) • Sound output port for recording/playback and attaching headphones or patch cable (3.5 mm mono) • <100+ amplification (caution is advised)
ThinkLabs ds32a+ Digital Stethoscope with ANR2 HC-TL/ STETH1	Amplified	• Ambient noise reduction • Audio input/output port • <100× amplification (caution is advised) • Available on the market, but discontinued by manufacturer (see ThinkLabs One)

Note. Amplification measures are relative to conventional nonamplified acoustic stethoscopes.

nonamplified stethoscope, calculations indicate that it comes to about a 33 dB SPL improvement. Table 14–3 shows how reported amplification values in SPL differ from power and loudness values for the same dB. Unless otherwise specified, manufacturers will use the SPL amplification factor. To illustrate example uses of amplified and visual stethoscopes, Figure 14–2 shows how four health professionals with hearing loss use their equipment.

For the audiologist who will modify the programming of hearing aids or implant devices for stethoscope use, the following suggestions are offered: Consider creating a dedicated program or MAP specific for stethoscope use. Have the stethoscope user describe and offer examples (real or simulated) of auscultation sounds that he or she will be expected to hear. Recall that many auscultation sounds will be below 1000 Hz, with some sounds extending down as low as 20 Hz. Fortunately, most auscultation sounds will be broadband in nature and will have signature characteristics in tim-

ing, frequency/energy spread, and timbre to improve detection and analysis. Except with special instrumentation, audiometers and probe microphone hearing aid fitting systems will not permit testing at very low frequencies. For example, most audiometers do not extend below 250 Hz, although some will extend down to 125 Hz. Likewise, most hearing aid fitting systems will not extend below 200 Hz as they were designed mainly for speech frequencies. Thus, subjective qualifications by the stethoscope user will be important. Consider the various options for coupling the stethoscope to the hearing aid or implant device, and recognize that the telecoil response using an induction neckloop or silhouette may be inadequate for very low frequencies. Since we will not know what the listener's hearing sensitivity is below 125 Hz, boosting the gain in the low frequencies may or may not be needed. As an example, a listener with severe-to-profound hearing loss may very well have normal or near normal thresholds below 125 Hz. Finally, it should be recalled that the hearing aid amplified frequency

Table 14–3. Relationship for Differences in Sound Pressure, Power, and Loudness for Changes in Decibel (dB)

Sound Pressure Level Difference	Power Difference	Loudness Difference	Decibel (dB)
10×	100×	4×	20.0 dB
16×	251×	5.3×	24.1 dB
24×	576×	6.8×	27.6 dB
50×	2500×	10.5×	33.9 dB
100×	10000×	16×	40.0 dB

Note. Calculations made through http://www.sengpielaudio.com/calculator-levelchange.htm

Figure 14–2. Examples of amplified and visual stethoscopes in use. **A.** Dr. Juan Esteban Lopez, veterinarian, using Cardionics E-Scope Hearing Impaired Model stethoscope coupled using direct-audio input (DAI) patch cord to behind-the-ear (BTE) hearing aid with audio shoe. Photo credit: Angela Novile. **B.** Dr. Danielle Rastetter, veterinarian, using ThinkLabs One stethoscope coupled to cochlear implant. Photo credit: Steven Knick. **C.** Amber Kimball, nurse, using Cardionics E-Scope with high-quality headphones placed over the hearing aid or cochlear implant. Photo credit: Chett DeLong. **D.** Dr. Megan Jack, physician, using Cardionics Vi-Scope Hearing Impaired Model, which also has audio output capabilities. Photo credit: Megan Jack.

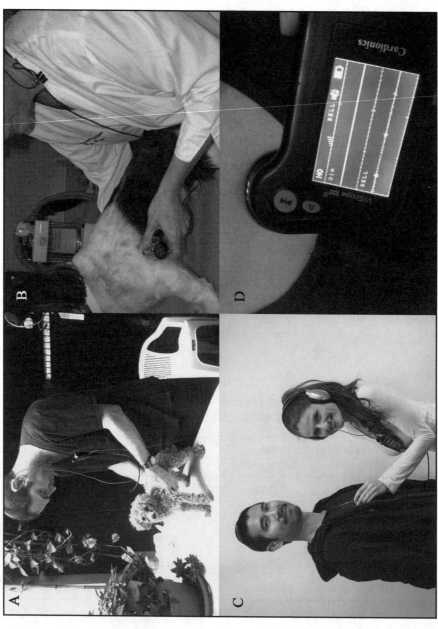

240

response gain and the low-frequency cut-off of cochlear implants may also be limiting factors at low frequencies. Although a hearing aid frequency response may extend below 200 Hz, one will not be able to measure this objectively with existing clinical systems. For cochlear implants, it has been reported that the low-frequency cutoff can vary across both make and model and will range anywhere between 75 and 200 Hz. Programming hearing aids and implant devices for higher-frequency auscultation sounds will likely be much easier.

Protective Face Masks

Depending on the severity of hearing loss and the amount of background noise, lipreading (or speechreading) is a helpful visual aid for spoken communication. One major barrier for health professionals (and patients) with hearing loss is communication with someone who is wearing a face mask. The most common face mask seen in health care is the disposable type made with three-ply/three-layer material that is pleated or folded, and it covers the mouth and nose. To hold the mask in place over the mouth and nose, tie straps, ear loops, or adhesives are used. The goal of these face masks is to prevent the spread of airborne diseases in the form of liquid droplets, and it has been demonstrated that this type of face mask does not impact the acoustic transmission of speech sounds through the material (Mendel, Gardino, & Atcherson, 2008). Some face masks have large plastic shields designed to be highly resistant to splashing liquid and body fluids. These face mask shields will come in one of two forms: (1) a lightweight shield that protects the face from splashes but offers no protection from airborne diseases and (2) a lightweight shield system that protects the face from splashes but is combined with a helmet and hood to protect the whole head and also offer protection from airborne diseases. An example of the shield system with helmet and hood is the Stryker® T5 Personal Protection System, which does not obscure the mouth. Unfortunately, the T5 system will not be cost effective, nor will it be appropriate for everyday, ordinary clinical tasks. When a face shield must be combined with a face mask, the mouth is obscured again.

Over the past 15 years, several prototypes of disposable see-through face masks have been proposed that use respiratory and splatter protection materials. However, because of the close proximity to the mouth and nose, these are often prone to fogging, and defeat the purpose of the face mask for communication. The only product that came to market but later became unavailable is a product made by Nex-Gen Clear Surgical Mask produced by SAM-GO back in 2011. The Nex-Gen mask was a modified oxygen mask with built-in filtration system. Although the mask was clear and was somewhat resistant to fogging, the filter and the light reflection off the surface of the oxygen mask were just enough to distort and obscure lipreading. Furthermore, the oxygen mask muffled speech sounds making it especially difficult for a person with hearing loss to understand what was said by the person wearing the respirator mask. Inventors Jeanne Hahne, RN, in San Francisco, California, and Gary Behm, Associate Professor of Engineering Studies in Rochester, New York, have each developed see-through face mask prototypes that look more like the conventional, disposable face masks. At the time of this writing, however, neither has moved to the production phase. Anecdotally, it has been reported that Kimberly-Clark Corporation is close to the production of a see-through mask based on the 1996 patent of inventor Gerald Carlson II (US Patent # US5561863 A). To have a face mask that is transparent, does not fog, and still offers respiratory and splatter protection would be a useful product. Such a product would benefit not only persons with hearing loss but also individuals with foreign accents, for situations when there is a lot of background noise, and to reduce anxiety by making the person wearing the mask more identifiable.

Alerting Systems

Some health professionals may need to monitor signals in the same work location but from different rooms. An overview of many alerting systems is described in Chapter 12, but here we highlight an example product system for this scenario. The Communicator receiver is one such product sold by Silent Call Communications (Figure 14–3). The Communicator is a wearable, portable vibration alert device. On the device are digital display icons to alert the wearer to sound, telephone, doorbell, weather alert, carbon monoxide alarm, fire alarm, and smoke detector alarm. For each of these signal types, there are separate transmitters that would need to be purchased. Interestingly, there are some additional transmitters that can be used without a specific display icon on the Communicator device, but substitutions are allowable. For example, there is a Bed Mat transmitter that can be placed under the bed sheet. The transmitter will send an alert to the Communicator device if the person lying on the bed mat gets up out of bed.

Designated Interpreters

Though not a technology per se, some health professionals and students with hearing loss use sign language interpreters for access to verbal and nonverbal auditory communication in the classroom, during training activities, and in the workforce. There may be one or two interpreters that aid the health professional or student in the translation of spoken language communication. They may continue to use other hearing assistive and access technologies to perform their work. Due to the specialized nature of the deaf professional (or aspiring deaf professional), interpreters in health care settings require specialized training as if they were also in the practice of that health profession. The term *designated interpreter* is appropriate here. Interpreters generally take a neutral approach to communication—that is, they are not active participants, but rather serve as conduits for communication (Napier, Carmichael, & Wiltshire, 2008). However, designated interpreters have long partnerships with the deaf professional, and they become

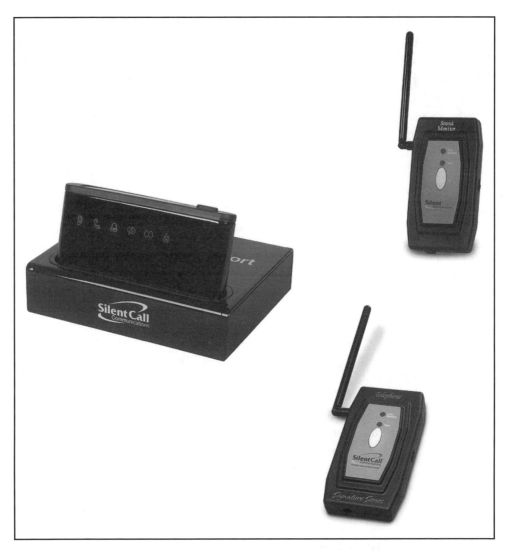

Figure 14–3. Example multiple transmitter alert system by Silent Call Communications with sound monitor and telephone transmitters. Images courtesy of Silent Call Communications.

part of the work environment and professional team (Hauser, Finch, & Hauser, 2008). There must occur a high level of mutual trust as the designated interpreter becomes the deaf professionals' ears (and sometimes eyes), and when appropriate, the deaf professionals' voice. This is quite difficult to do if the neutral conduit approach is taken. Interested readers are directed to the edited work of Hauser, Finch, and Hauser (2008) to learn more about the deaf professional-designated interpreter model. As an example, professional interpreter Lani Crosby spent the last two years of Michael McKee, MD's medical training assisting him in the operating room and on rounds (Arndorfer, 2001). During the last year, Crosby was on call whenever needed and spent time during off-hours studying the medical terminology that would be critical to communicate with patients. Beyond medical school, Christopher Moreland, MD, MPH, continues to use a team of designated interpreters, Todd Agan and Keri Richardson, when he communicates with his patients, with colleagues, and with medical residents and students (Henkel, 2014). One would wonder what patients might feel with the interpreter in the room. Dr. Moreland experimented with different approaches and the one that appeared to put the patient most at ease was simply introducing himself and his interpreter briefly, and then focusing back on the patient to develop rapport and trust. Although the examples shown here involve physicians, similar designated interpreter arrangements have been made in other fields.

Spotlight: Audiologists With Hearing Loss

Audiologists are allied health professionals who deal with hearing and balance disorders. Audiology is predominantly a sound-based field, which offers unique challenges when the audiologist has hearing loss (Atcherson & Spangler, 2014; Yoder & Pratt, 2005). Aside from having potential hearing-related challenges in the classroom and during clinical training with patients, the two biggest challenges that cause the most anxiety involve speech recognition testing and the analysis and troubleshooting of hearing aids and implant device components. Some solutions are offered below for these two areas. A third challenge for some audiologists with hearing loss is communication with their patients during appointments and communication over the telephone. Solutions for these are offered elsewhere in this book, but it is important to note that all audiologists, including those with hearing loss, have an incredible opportunity to teach and model to patients about advocacy, communication strategies, and technologies beyond hearing aids and implant devices in order to promote independence and a satisfactory quality of life. To this point, if an audiologist with hearing loss must use a hearing assistive device such as an FM system or 2.4 GHz remote microphone system during appointments with patients, this is a powerful teaching moment. Finally, audiologists with hearing loss often wonder whether or not they should disclose their own hearing loss to patients. There is no best answer for whether or not to disclose, but the best thing an audiologist with hearing loss can do is demonstrate good communication and listening behaviors, confidence, competence, and professionalism. There is no doubt that sharing one's own hearing loss story may help a patient gain insights into his or her own problems, but an audiologist should make sure that the majority of the appointment time remains focused on the patient.

Speech Recognition When the Audiologist Has Hearing Loss

Audiologists with hearing loss are acutely aware of their own speech recognition abilities. As the severity of hearing loss increases, speech recognition abilities become poorer. However, as reported by Han, Schlauch, and Rao (2014), speech recognition performance recorded by all audiologists (hearing loss or not) is subject to error. However, the audiologist with hearing loss must ensure that his or her hearing loss is minimized as a contributing factor. An audiologist with hearing loss will have some advantages that the patient will not have. For example, the audiologist with hearing loss may be able to take advantage of visual cues by lipreading the patient during speech recognition testing. This is confirmed by Han et al. for all audiologists. To see the patient better, the audiologist with hearing loss might consider turning off or dimming the lights on the examiner side. Sound booths are often not sufficiently bright and have lights directly above the patient, which can cast a shadow on the patient's face. A small light source placed in front of the patient may help brighten the patient's face to allow lipreading. If the audiometer talkback system is not sufficient to hear patient verbal responses, the audiologist with hearing loss could use an FM system (Schutzenhofer, 2009) or remote microphone system and place a microphone directly on or near the patient. With some patients, it may be necessary to have patients write down what they heard, either because lipread-ing is difficult, because speech is difficult to understand (even for normal listeners), or because of an accent. A major drawback is that some patients may lack the ability to write or may have poor spelling (Francart, Moonen, & Wouters, 2009; Han et al., 2014). Han et al. also suggest having some patients put the word in a sentence. Both methods, however, are time consuming. With respect to the presentation of speech stimuli, monitored live voice speech should be avoided, especially if the audiologist's own voice and articulation are not typical.

Listening To a Patient's Hearing Aids and Implantable Devices

In contrast to listening to auscultation sounds, audiologists may use an acoustic stethoscope, often called a listening scope or stethoset, to listen to the quality of their patient's hearing aids. Monaural listening scopes can be used with a standard rubber ear tip to place into the ear canal, or they can be personalized with a custom earmold. At the end of either the monaural or binaural listening scope is a rubber bell (or hollow bulb) used to attach the receiver end of a hearing aid earhook, earmold, or dome. If the patient's unaided hearing is similar to the audiologist's unaided hearing, a listening scope could be used. Figure 14–1 shows how one audiologist with hearing loss uses her listening scope with Westone Stethocut custom earmolds. In this case, no additional amplification is required, and she does not have to take her own hearing aids out. However, if the audiologist's unaided hearing is worse than that of the patient, some additional amplification would be required. Either the signal must be amplified into the unaided audiologist's ear, or the signal must be routed into the audiologist's own hearing aid or implant device.

Figure 14–4 shows two listening scopes using sacrificed stethoset parts. The Starkey ST3 stethoscope was a clever device designed for auscultation, but it also had a built-in hearing aid. In this figure, the bell and diaphragm of the ST3 were replaced with a stethoset bulb to permit listening to other hearing aids. For this modified stethoset to work, the output of the patient's hearing aid fed acoustically into stethoscope's built-in microphone, amplifier, and receiver system, which was converted back into an acoustic signal. Thus, the ST3 built-in amplifier served as the audiologist's hearing aid. The battery-powered RadioShack

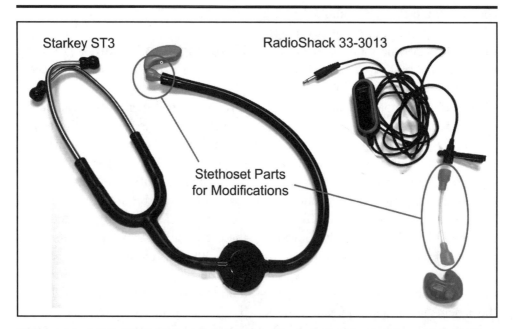

Figure 14–4. Modified stethoset examples for audiologists with hearing loss. *Left:* A Starkey ST3 amplified stethoscope (discontinued, but may be available secondhand) was modified by replacing the standard chestpiece for heart and lung auscultation with a stethoset earmold bell to listen to hearing aids. In order to use the Starkey ST3, however, the user has to remove his/her own hearing aids or use a Westone Stethocut earmold shown in Figure 14–1. *Right:* A RadioShack 33-3013 lavalier microphone was outfitted with stethoset parts (two earmold bells and tubing) to listen to hearing aids. The 3.5-mm jack can then be used as a direct audio input (DAI) to personal hearing devices or amplifiers (e.g., Streamer, FM transmitter/receiver system, etc.). Reprint permission from the American Academy of Audiology.

33-3013 lavalier microphone has stethoset parts on the end of the microphone. The microphone immediately accepts the output of the patient's hearing aid, but now the audiologist has one of several choices from which to connect the microphone (e.g., DAI, Streamer, FM system, portable amplifier, a computer amplifier, etc.).

A much more elaborate setup to boost gain and permit Bluetooth transmission to the audiologist's Bluetooth-enabled hearing aids is offered in Figure 14–5. Here, in addition to the RadioShack 33-3013 lavalier microphone, a RadioShack Mini Audio Amplifier is added midstream to provide greater gain. A patch cable is used to connect the RadioShack Mini Audio Amplifier to a Phonak ComPilot, which will then be used to send the signal wirelessly to hearing aids or implant devices capable of receiving the ComPilot signal.

Although there may be many other approaches, at least one more is offered here for listening to a patient's hearing aid: If the audiologist has access to a probe microphone system, such as the Audioscan Verifit hearing aid test box, a headphone jack is available to allow any audiologist to listen to the output of the patient's hearing aid while it is connected to the 2-cc coupler. The audiologist with hearing loss now has one of several options using the headphone jack. Figure 14–6 shows a bilateral cochlear implant user with a pair of headphones while the cochlear implants are set to telecoil mode. If all else fails, a hearing aid test box will always be a useful tool in troubleshooting hearing aids.

Audiologists may also have tools available to listen to the microphone of cochlear implants or to the output of a bone-anchored hearing device. There are plenty of strategies indicated above that might help audiologists with hearing loss listen through their own hearing aid or implant device, which will depend on the coupling option available. A conversation with the implant device manufacturer may also be worthwhile to consider additional strategies or modifications.

Summary

Individuals with hearing loss should no longer be barred from careers in health care. Granted, prospective students will still need to meet the academic and technical standards for the program. Specific to individuals with hearing loss, students will need to ensure that communication and alternative access to job-related sounds can be achieved reliably. Health professionals with hearing loss well into their careers would do well to keep up with the latest in hearing assistive and access technology to continue to maintain and advance their clinical skills and competencies. For interested readers, there are a number of recommended resources to continue the topic of health professionals with hearing loss (e.g., Maheady, 2003; Morris, 2007; Task Force on Health Care Careers for the Deaf and Hard-of-Hearing Community, 2012).

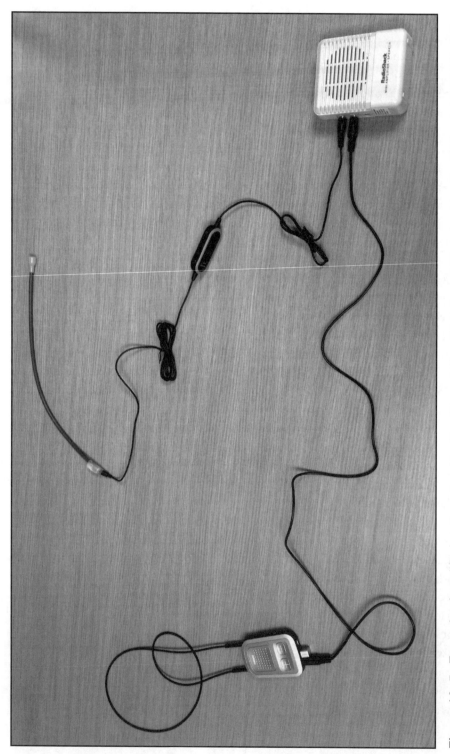

Figure 14–5. Example of modified stethoset used with a Phonak ComPilot. For additional gain, a RadioShack 33-3013 lavalier microphone was paired with a RadioShack Mini Audio Amplifier. A patch cord was used to connect the external audio jack of the RadioShack Amplifier to the Phonak ComPilot. Photo credit: Andrew Couch, AuD.

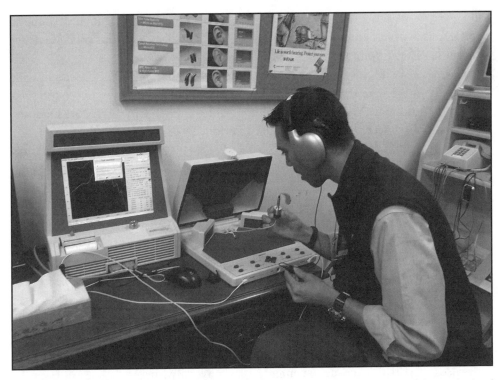

Figure 14–6. Example of a hearing aid listening check using the headphone jack of the Audioscan Verifit hearing aid fitting system. The headphones can be used acoustically or via telecoil on the audiologist's own hearing aids or cochlear implant. The headphones have a built-in amplifier to offer additional gain, if necessary. Photo credit: Kimberlee Crass, PhD.

References

Argenyi v. Creighton University, 703 F.3d 441 (8th Cir. 2013).

Arndorfer, B. (2001, May 26). Silencing doubters. *Gainesville Sun*.

Atcherson, S. R., & Spangler, C. (2014, Mar/Apr). Functionally the same, yet different: Audiologists with hearing loss. *Audiology Today, 26*(2), 42–48.

Busch-Vishniac, I. J., West, J. E., Barnhill, C., Hunter, T., Orellana, D., & Chivukula, R. (2005). Noise levels in Johns Hopkins Hospital. *Journal of the Acoustical Society of America, 118*(6), 3629–3645.

Clark III, D., Ahmed, M. I., Dell'Italia, L. J., Fan, P., & McGiffin, D. C. (2012). An argument for reviving the disappearing skill of cardiac auscultation. *Cleveland Clinic Journal of Medicine, 79*(8), 536–544.

Dietrich S. (2005). Road Test: An FM system in a dental office/educational setting. *Hearing Review, 12*(1), 38–42.

Falk, S. A., & Woods, N. F. (1973). Hospital noise—levels and potential noise hazards. *New England Journal of Medicine, 289,* 774–781.

Francart, T., Moonen, M., & Wouters, J. (2009). Automatic testing of speech recognition. *International Journal of Audiology, 48*(2), 80–90.

Han, H. J., Schlauch, R. S., & Rao, A. (2014). The effect of visual cues on scoring of clinical word-recognition tests. *American Journal of Audiology, 23*(4), 385–393.

Hauser, P. C., Finch, K. L., & Hauser, A. B. (Eds.). (2008). *Deaf professionals and designated interpreters: A new paradigm* (Vol. 3). Washington, DC: Gallaudet University Press.

Henkel, G. (2014, August). Deaf hospitalist focuses on teaching, co-management, patient-centered care. *The Hospitalist.* Retrieved from http://www.the-hospitalist.org/details/article/6443271/ Deaf_Hospitalist_Focuses_on_Teaching _Co-Management_Patient-Centered_ Care.html

Larkin, M. (2009). Deaf veterinarians pave their own way. *Journal of the American Veterinary Association, 235*(10), 1120–1123.

Maheady, D. C. (2003). *Nursing with disabilities: Change the course.* River Edge, NJ: Exceptional Parent Press.

Mendel, L. L., Gardino, J. A., & Atcherson, S. R. (2008). Speech understanding using surgical masks: A problem in health care? *Journal of the American Academy of Audiology, 19*(9), 686–695.

Moreland, C. J., Latimore, D., Sen, A., Arato, N., & Zazove, P. (2013). Deafness among physicians and trainees: A national survey. *Academic Medicine, 88*(2), 224–232.

Morris, R. (2007). *On the job with hearing loss: Hidden challenges. Successful solutions.* Garden City, NY: Morgan James.

Perloff, D., Grim, C., Flack, J., Frohlich, E. D., Hill, M., McDonald, M., & Morgenstern, B. Z. (1993). Human blood pressure determination by sphygmomanometry. *Circulation, 88,* 2460–2470.

Napier, J., Carmichael, A., & Wiltshire, A. (2008). Look-pause-nod: A linguistic case study of a Deaf professional and interpreters working together. In P. C. Hauser, K. L. Finch, & A. B. Hauser (Eds.), *Deaf professionals and designated interpreters: A new paradigm* (pp. 22–42). Washington, DC: Gallaudet University Press.

Rhodes, R. S., Davis, D. C., & Odom, B. C. (1999). Challenges and rewards of educating a profoundly deaf student. *Nurse Educator, 24*(3), 48–51.

Schutzenhofer, S. (2009). *Utilizing hearing assistive technology (HAT) to assess speech recognition: Comparison of word recognition scores obtained by hearing instrument users. (AuD capstone).* Retrieved from http://digitalcommons. wustl.edu/pacs_capstones/399

Task Force on Health Care Careers for the Deaf and Hard-of-Hearing Community. (2012). *Building pathways to health care careers for the deaf and hard-of-hearing community.* Retrieved from http://www.rit.edu/ntid/hccd/ reports

Velde, B. P., Chapin, M. H., & Wittman, P. P. (2005). Working around "it": The experience of occupational therapy students with a disability. *Journal of Allied Health, 34*(2), 83–89.

Yoder, S., & Pratt, S. (2005). Audiologists who have hearing loss: Demographics and specific accommodation needs. *Journal of the Academy of Rehabilitative Audiology, 38,* 11–29.

15

What's New at the Zoo? Recent Advances in Technology

Overview

The use of hearing aids, implantable devices, frequency-modulated (FM) systems, soundfield amplification systems, infrared (IR) systems, induction hearing loop systems, and other hearing assistive and access technologies are generally well established, but they often remain underused due to lack of awareness, lack of understanding, or financial constraints. Depending on one's view, this issue could become better or worse as hearing assistive and access technologies (1) become obsolete in favor of a newer technology (2) evolve in size, shape, and manner of use; and (3) are newly conceived, implemented, and marketed. The goal of hearing assistive and access technologies is to help create a world in which individuals with hearing loss have equal opportunities with regard to this otherwise sound-based world, with the majority of its citizens having normal hearing. Unless adequate prevention measures are taken, hearing loss in many individuals will be inevitable due to continued loud noise exposure, age-related hearing loss, poor health-related habits, and genetic determinants. Hearing assistive and access technologies may well benefit individuals with hearing loss, but in many cases, they have also benefited people with normal hearing (e.g., telephone invented by A. G. Bell and the acoustic modem invented by R. H. Weitbrecht, J. C. Marsters, and A. Saks). Likewise, individuals with hearing loss may benefit from technologies designed for the masses (e.g., electronic and digital text messaging and e-mail), a positive side effect.

This final chapter focuses not only on new and soon-to-be-released technology, but also on some creative uses of new or existing technology. Some of these technologies have been introduced in the preceding chapters, but we bring them to the forefront again in this chapter because they are so new, they represent the current state of the art, and they will shape the future. The first part of this chapter touches on innovation and creativity related to hearing aids and implantable devices, such as remote microphones. The remaining portion of the chapter focuses on invention and creativity not specifically related to hearing aids or implantable devices. With technology changing as rapidly as it does, the information presented in this chapter may soon be obsolete. Therefore, it is the innovative application, as well as the innovative technology, that may be gleaned from this chapter with an eye toward the future.

Technology Related to Hearing Aids and Implantable Devices

Remote Microphones

One of the chief complaints from hearing aid wearers has been listening and understanding in the presence of background noise. With the use of remote microphones such as Phonak's Roger Pen (see Figure 4–10), as a hearing aid accessory, noise between the speaker and the hearing aid wearer can be greatly reduced. The remote microphone is simply placed near the speaker's mouth as he or she speaks and the signal is transmitted directly to the hearing aids. The speaker can hold the remote microphone, clip it to an article of clothing, or hang it on a loop around the neck. Because the speaker's voice does not have to travel through the air and suffer the effects of the Inverse Square Law (see Chapter 3), and will not be negatively affected by either background noise or reverberation, the signal-to-noise (SNR) ratio is considerably better than hearing aids alone, even with directional microphones engaged on the hearing aids.

Digital Enhanced Cordless Telecommunications Telephones

Communicating over a telephone has been quite a challenge for those with hearing loss as no visual cues are provided and telephone filters limit the frequency range available. Using a common landline telephone requires the signal to be converted from an electronic signal to an acoustic signal and back. The chance of interference increases with each of these conversions. In addition, the interaction between telephone and hearing aid often results in a distortion of the hearing aid's amplified signal, known as feedback. Feedback, usually indicated by a squeal or whistle from the hearing aid, causes many hearing aid wearers to stop using the telephone. The digital enhanced cordless telecommunications (DECT) telephones introduced in Chapter 9 transmit the signal directly to both hearing aids. There is no need for conversion between the telephone and the hearing aids. Therefore, there is minimal interference and no feedback. Also, allowing hearing aid wearers to listen with both ears provides a sizable advantage over listening with only one ear. Using DECT telephones can significantly decrease listening effort, increase sound quality and overall impression, and assist in finding the best hearing aid receiver position (Latzel & Appleton-Huber, 2013). Presently, DECT telephones are compatible only with some hearing aids. Similar effects can be found in the communication between hearing aids and smartphones via Bluetooth.

Wireless Communication Between Hearing Aids

Directional microphones have been in use for decades and improve the SNR for hearing aid wearers. Although bilateral wireless communication between hearing aids (see Chapter 4) is now a commonly used technology, it is innovative as two sets of directional microphones, two microphones from each of the two hearing aids, can be combined to provide an even greater SNR. The hearing aid wearer's head causes a difference in sound intensity levels between the hearing aids, known as the *head-shadow effect.* This difference in intensity between the hearing aids allows the four microphones to better minimize the noise processed in each hearing aid, resulting in an improved SNR.

Wireless Communication With Smart Devices

Smart devices have the ability to transmit and receive signals to and from other devices such as hearing aids (see Chapters 4 and 9). Using a smart device and a streaming device, hearing aids can receive signals from smartphones, MP3 players, computers, televisions, and other devices with minimal interference from background noise. Generally, overall satisfaction with hearing aids use improves with the increased number of listening situations in which the hearing aids are considered useful (Kochkin, 2011). In addition, as with the use of DECT phones, the signal can be transmitted to both hearing aids. Hearing aid wearers can also use the microphone on a smart device as a remote microphone by simply pairing the smart device with the hearing aids and the appropriate application on the smart device.

Some hearing aids have the ability to communicate with smart devices without the need of a streaming device. Again, communication with other devices provides hearing aid wearers the ability to hear the signal in both ears, and allows the microphone on a smart device to be used as a remote microphone. When hearing aids communicate directly with smart devices, no streamer is needed, resulting in one less device to keep track of and maintain. Also, direct communication between the hearing aids and smart device allows the smart device to act as a remote control in adjusting the hearing aids.

Wireless technology is not limited to applications with hearing aids. Implantable devices and personal sound amplification products (PSAPs) also have wireless communication capabilities (see Chapter 4). It is understandable that implantable devices, being relatively recent advances in hearing assistance technology, would lag behind the technologically competitive hearing aid industry in implementing contemporary wireless technology (e.g., Bluetooth). However, cochlear implant devices have recently employed such technology to open new doors for those with implants. Now, many cochlear implant recipients have the ability to receive signals directly from Bluetooth-enabled devices such as smartphones, televisions, MP3 players, computers, iPads, and so forth. A marketing image in Figure 15–1 illustrates some of the applications available via contemporary wireless technology.

Technology Not Directly Related to Hearing Aids and Implantable Devices

Emergency Management and Notification Services

Having a life or death emergency to deal with is a scary event for anyone. If there is access to a telephone or mobile phone, a 911 call can be placed for emergency assistance. For individuals with hearing loss, there can be greater anxiety because of the increased time needed to place the call through nontraditional means in order to reach emergency authorities. Mobile devices, teletypewriters (TTY), captioned telephones, and videophones can all be used in cases of emergency. However, since we cannot always predict where we will be and in what kind of situation (e.g., physical injury and without hearing aids or implant at the time of the emergency), these methods of calling for assistance may not be successful. This is especially true if one dials 911 and is unable to carry on a conversation with the emergency operator. In some cases, the emergency operator has the technology to pinpoint your location. Although there are many options for letting others know about an emergency, two examples using newer technologies are discussed here. The first is the use of the Smart911 service. This is a national database emergency system and an enhancement of existing 911 services. It is completely voluntary to participate in this national

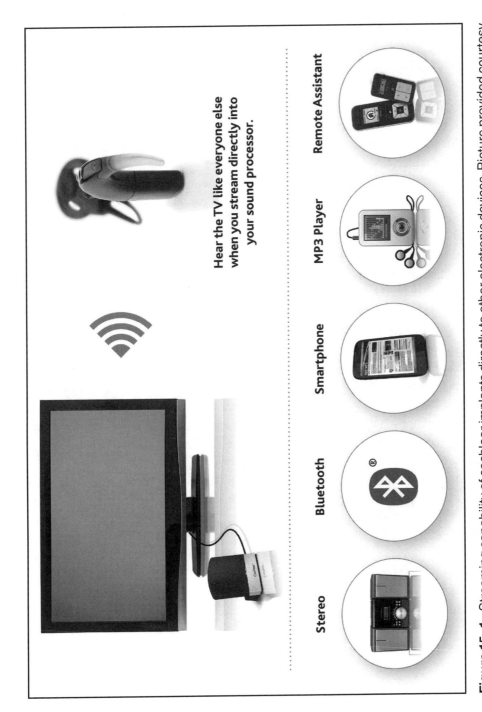

Hear the TV like everyone else when you stream directly into your sound processor.

Stereo Bluetooth Smartphone MP3 Player Remote Assistant

Figure 15–1. Streaming capability of cochlear implants directly to other electronic devices. Picture provided courtesy of Cochlear Americas, © 2014 Cochlear Americas.

database and communities will have the service only if they elect to use it. If the Smart911 service is in place, individuals with disabilities can register their personal information helpful for emergency operators to know. For example, the safety profile provided by the registrant could have information about the number of people in residence, floor plans, and other rescue-related data. For individuals with hearing loss who are unable to communicate, a call to 911 from a registered number would trigger the safety profile of the caller, and the emergency operator would have specific information for emergency responders. Smart911 may also allow emergency operators to engage in a text messaging (short message service; SMS) session with the caller. More information about this service can be found at http://www.smart911.com/

The second is taking advantage of one of several apps, aptly named "emergency button" or "panic button." The idea behind these apps is for users to preconfigure messages to specific individuals in case of an emergency. Using the cellular service, Wi-Fi, and GPS, messages may be sent indicating the emergency and give GPS coordinates of the individual's whereabouts. Reviews of the various apps are mixed because of the sensitivity of the button and the accuracy of the alert. However, all agree that these apps could be very useful but could benefit from improvement and refinement. Such technology would be useful to individuals both with and without hearing loss.

Video Calling: Not Just for Distant Communication

When listening environments involve a significant distance between the speaker and the listener, hampering the use of visual cues, use of a video projection system can facilitate the use of visual information. Because visual cues can supplement hearing, many lecture halls, worship centers, boardrooms, and other facilities have projection systems that can easily project the image of the speaker onto a screen to help the audience. With or without hearing loss, visual cues make listening easier. Figure 15–2 illustrates the use of video projection in a moderate-sized classroom, while Figure 15–3 represents a large lecture hall.

When a facility does not have a video projection system or a camera, video calling may, in the near future, become a viable substitute for a projection system. If the speaker has a smart device with a camera, the video, along with the audio, can be transmitted to other smart devices around the world, or to the back of the room. Presently, application of this technology is limited by the relatively low number of smart devices than can receive the video call. Also, there is a small, but significant, time delay between the transmission and reception of the signal, which could compromise the synchrony of the auditory and visual signals.

Video calling technology includes combining audio and video transmissions, but in relatively close proximity to the transmitting device, such as within

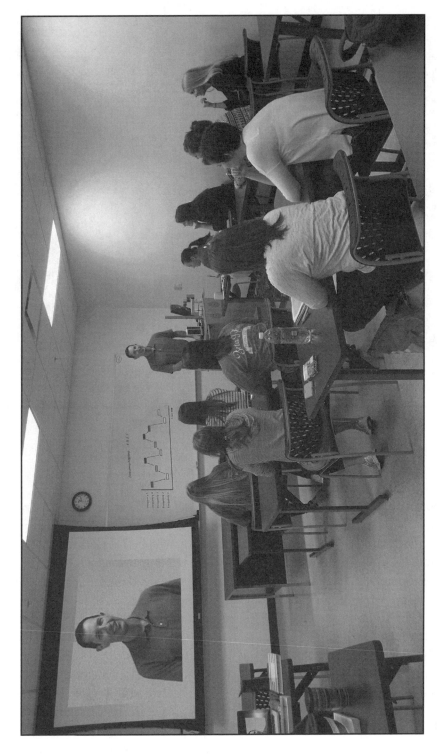

Figure 15–2. Use of video projection to facilitate use of visual cues in a moderate-sized classroom. Photo credit: Samuel R. Atcherson, PhD.

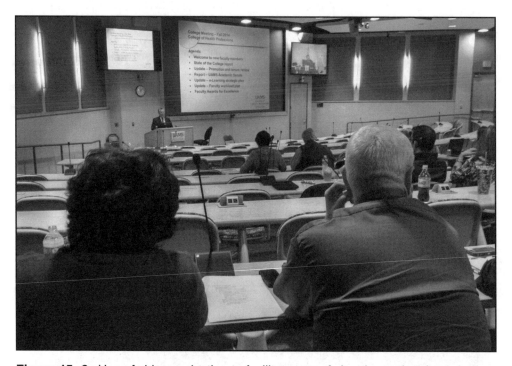

Figure 15–3. Use of video projection to facilitate use of visual cues in a large lecture hall. Photo credit: Clifford A. Franklin, PhD.

a large lecture hall. Applications of this popular technology include FaceTime, Skype, ooVoo, and Google Plus Hangouts. While these applications are similar in that they allow rapid transmission of both audio and video data, there are differences. Some applications may use videotelephony, while others may use Voice over Internet Protocol (VoIP), which is dependent on access to a Wi-Fi signal. The time delay between transmission and reception, previously mentioned, and issues related to video clarity may decrease in importance with recent Wi-Fi transmission speeds increasing to 60 GHz.

Doorbells

For those with hearing loss, hearing a doorbell can be an invisible challenge, as the person with hearing loss may not realize there was ever anyone at the door. Some doorbell systems designed for those with hearing loss allow strobe lights or lamps inside the house to flash when the doorbell button is pressed. Doorbells using modern wireless technology can also improve this situation, as the receiving device (i.e., the bell) can be carried and placed in the same room or area of the house as the resident, or, multiple receivers may be used. These systems are not "new to the zoo," but some newer doorbells are designed to work with a Wi-Fi system to send the signal to a smart device. Not only can the resident be alerted via multiple smart devices located throughout the home, but they can also receive video from a small camera mounted in the button. For the "do-it-yourselfer," a common doorbell can be connected to the base of a DECT phone system's "find handset" feature. With the base capable of communicating with multiple handsets, the beeping handset/receivers are more likely to be heard. Although many of us would prefer to purchase a manufactured doorbell system, a system can be constructed with a bit of technical knowledge and creative savvy.

Bed Vibration Alert Device

Although bed vibration alert devices are not new, inventors and cofounders of Cenify, Alex Satterly and Patrick Seypura, are deaf and taking advantage of the Internet of Things (IoT) to simplify life with smart-home devices. Soon to be available, a bed vibration device, the Alarmify, is triggered by a smartphone alarm clock app. While a smartphone has vibration capabilities, it is generally not strong enough and placing a smartphone between the mattress and box spring or in a pillowcase negates the other functions of the smartphone.

Intercom System

A common complaint from those with hearing loss and their family and friends is the difficulty understanding what is spoken when shouting from one room of the house to the next. When trying to communicate from one room to another, the best practice is for the two individuals to come into close proximity of one another to minimize the challenges of distance and reverberation. However, for some reason, we as speakers and listeners almost invariably tend to try the shouting method, only to become frustrated. Intercom systems can facilitate communication from one part of a building or house to another. Traditional intercom systems require preplanning or construction work to include running wire through walls, ceilings, and/or floors. One alternative is to use the "push to talk" and/or the "speaker phone" feature(s) to make a set of DECT telephones function as an intercom system. These telephones even allow simultaneous transmission between two or more phones, allowing both ends to speak and be heard at the same time. Some phone systems can function as an intercom without the need of holding the phone. Figure 15–4 provides an idea of how a DECT telephone system may be distributed around a house to be used as an intercom system, as well as a telephone system.

Open Ear Headphones

Most of us have a good understanding about sound moving through the air and reaching our ears. We may even know how the middle ear functions. But the inner ear contains the sensory organ named the

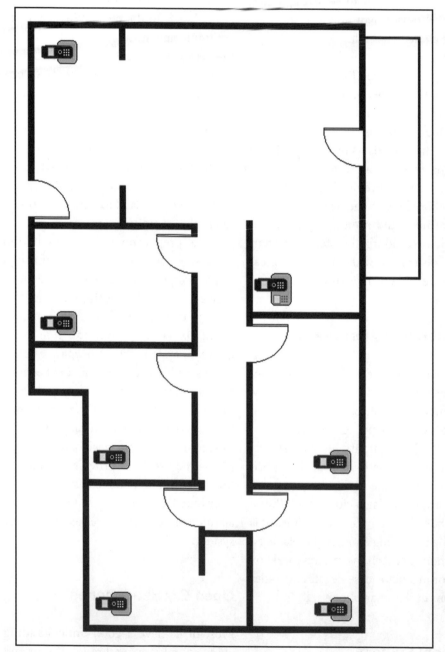

Figure 15–4. Cordless telephones using DECT technology can be arranged as an intercom system throughout the house.

Organ of Corti. Sound energy reaches the inner ear through the air, the outer ear, and the middle ear, known as hearing via *air conduction*. But sound energy can also reach the inner ear by vibrating the skull, referred to as hearing via *bone conduction*. The idea of placing a vibrating device against the head to vibrate the skull, and ultimately the inner ear, has been the foundation of bone conduction hearing aids for years. Recently, this technology has carried over to headphones, as bone conduction headphones have become available for purchase. These headphones allow the user to listen to MP3 players, computers, television, and so on, without blocking the air conduction pathway for hearing, and thus reducing the interference associated with such blockage. These bone conduction headphones may be worn while involved in outdoor activities such as running or cycling, in which it is critically important to hear environ-

mental sounds like oncoming traffic or sirens. These devices, called Aftershokz, connect directly to the audio output ports of most devices including mobile phones (Figure 15–5). Newer Bluetooth-enabled models, Bluez 2, allow for the same function without the cumbersome wire connection. More information may be obtained at http://www.aftershokz.com/

Other headphones transmit sound via air conduction but allow for the ear to remain open. Like the bone conduction headphones, this technology allows the wearer to listen to music while still being able to hear sounds in the environment. More information about these open ear headphones can be found at http://www.earhero.com/. Although these devices are not designed specifically for those with hearing loss, they may nonetheless be of benefit to some individuals with hearing loss without having to occlude the ear canals.

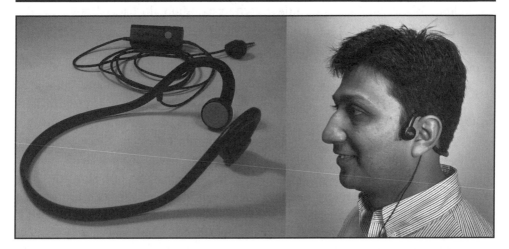

Figure 15–5. Open ear, bone conduction, headphones that allow the wearer to hear by way of vibrations directly stimulating the inner ear. Photo credit: Clifford A. Franklin, PhD.

Hearing Assistance With Google Glass

Google Glass is a smart device that is worn on the head in a structure designed to be worn much like that of common eyeglasses. These wearable computers offer interactive controls for features which include video/camera operations, local memory storage, wireless connectivity via Bluetooth and Wi-Fi, and bone conduction audio. Like bone conduction headphones, Google Glass audio does not block sounds from entering the ear, while providing sound, by way of bone conduction, to the inner ear. Even though these devices are not designed as hearing assistive technology, they may benefit those with hearing loss. In addition to the use of bone conduction audio transmission, Google Glass may help individuals with hearing loss by taking advantage of the glass for the projection of live, automatic, and pre-scripted captions, subtitles, and manual interpretation. The possibilities for Google Glass are endless. Additional information about Google Glass can be found at https://www.google.com/glass

Smart Apps

Downloadable applications, or *apps*, for smart devices can assist those with hearing loss. There are too many possible applications related to hearing assistance and access to be covered in this text. Therefore, this section merely introduces a few apps that may provide a starting point in the search for apps that fit a specific need.

First are amplifier apps, which receive sound via the microphone of the smart device, amplify the signal, and then deliver a more intense sound via internal or external speaker, or via headphones. Many of these apps are free but typically have a noticeable delay; however, some apps have significantly reduced the delay issue.

Bluetooth microphone apps, like amplifier apps, start with the microphone, but the signal is transmitted to an output device via Bluetooth instead of going to the smart device's speaker. Any Bluetooth-enabled device can be paired with the transmitting device to become part of a piconet (see Chapter 9).

As previously mentioned in the Intercom System section, trying to communicate from one room to the next is best facilitated by the two individuals coming closer to one another. Yet, speakers and listeners will almost always choose to shout, instead of moving to the same room. Bluetooth speakers, when strategically positioned, can become part of a system that allows for clearer communication between rooms, compared to shouting. Presently, there are better methods to deal with the challenges of communication in these situations, like the use of intercom systems (see the Intercom System section). Similarly, there are "walkie-talkie" apps that transform a smart device into a "walkie-talkie." As this technology is improved it may become more applicable to these challenges in the future.

Two speech-to-text apps have surfaced in the last year, one currently available and the other likely to be released in the near future. The ISeeWhatYouSay app (http://www.digitalarmydevices.com/) is an Android-based app available now and uses automatic speech recognition (ASR) in conjunction with wearable watch devices, such as the Bluetooth-enabled Pebble Watch (https://getpebble.com/) and the Android Wear (http://www.android.com/intl/en_us/wear/). As a person speaks into the smartphone, the text is displayed on the watch. The not-yet-available app that is generating excitement is another speech-to-text app incorporating ASR called Transcense (http://www.transcense.com/). The exact details of this app are not yet available, but it purports to be able to assist with group conversations.

Other apps may be useful in measuring a listening environment. Sound level measures and reverberation time are measurements usually conducted by dedicated, highly sensitive, and regularly calibrated sound level meters (SLMs). Sound level meters can be expensive and intimidating. However, for less accurate but still useful information, several smart device apps are available. Accuracy is mixed among SLM apps, and readers are encouraged to check out recent work by Huth, Popelka, and Blevins (2014), Nast, Speer, and Le Prell (2004), and Kardous and Shaw (2004). Figure 15–6 shows screenshots of a couple of SLM apps for smart devices. These apps may be of value when trying to acoustically improve a room. For example, measurements of sound

intensity and RT_{60} measures of reverberation can be conducted with these apps before and after the placement of sound-absorbing materials to provide an estimate of the efficacy of the acoustic treatment.

Summary

In this chapter, we briefly touched on topics of innovative technology related to and separate from hearing aids and implantable devices. Remote microphone technology, wireless communication between hearing aids and cochlear implants and smart devices was mentioned, as these technologies provide the listener with a direct signal and create a multitude of new listening experiences.

New technology discussed in this chapter, separate from that directly applicable to hearing aids and implantable devices, included alerting systems, such as doorbells and the valuable Smart911 service. Other topics in this chapter included the use of smart device apps, like SLMs and reverberation apps, to estimate changes in acoustic environments.

Even though this chapter is the final chapter of the textbook, and introduces many new and innovative technologies, it should not be viewed as an end of the information and technology available to those with hearing loss. Rather, this chapter, along with the other chapters in this book, should provide a foundation for further exploration into the best methods of gaining assistance for and access to better hearing and communication.

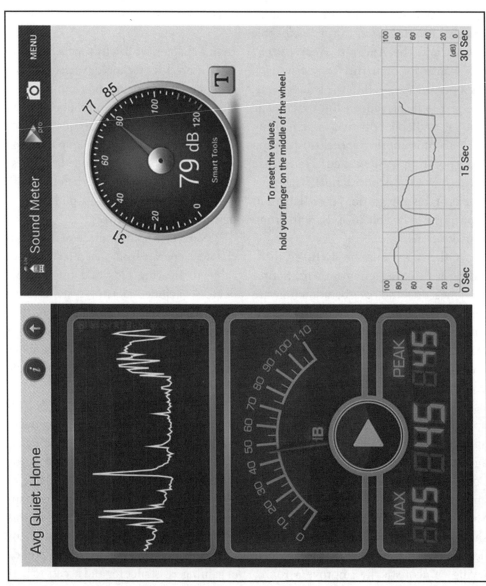

Figure 15–6. Smart device apps allow users to measure sound intensity and reverberation times for better assessment of listening environments. Photo credit: Clifford A. Franklin, PhD.

References

Huth, M. E., Popelka, G. R., & Blevins, N. H. (2014). Comprehensive measures of sound exposures in cinemas using smart phones. *Ear and Hearing, 35*(6), 680–686.

Kardous, C. A., & Shaw, P. B. (2014). Evaluation of smartphone sound measurement applications. *JASA Express Letters, 135*(4), EL186EL192.

Kochkin, S. (2011). MarkeTrak VIII: Patients report improved quality of life with hearing aid usage. *The Hearing Journal, 64*(6), 25–32.

Latzel, M., & Appleton-Huber, J. (2013). Improvement of speech intelligibility and subjective satisfaction with the new Phonak DECT cordless phone. *Audiologyonline*, Article 12223. Retrieved from http://www.audiologyonline.com

Nast, D. R., Speer, W. S., & Le Prell, C. G. (2014). Sound level measurement using smartphone "apps": Useful or inaccurate? *Noise and Health, 16*(72), 251–256.

Glossary

2.4 GHz Technology. See *Industrial, Scientific, and Medical (ISM) Frequency Band.*

Absorption Coefficients. Indication of how much sound is absorbed by a material.

Acceptable Noise Level (ANL). Defined as the maximum level of background noise that an individual is willing to accept while listening to speech.

Access. To make contact with or gain access to; be able to reach, approach, enter. In the case of a disability, access is synonymous with equal access, but not necessarily equal outcomes.

Accommodation. The process of adapting or adjusting to someone or something; a convenient arrangement, settlement, or compromise.

Acoustic Coupling. Describes the use of a microphone in hearing aids and implantable devices to pick up the transmission of speech and other desirable sounds via air conduction.

Activity Limitations. A difficulty encountered by an individual in executing a task or action.

Advocacy. Self or public support for, or recommendation of, a particular cause, policy, or need.

Air Conduction. Conduction of sound waves to the inner ear through the ear canal and middle ear.

Alerting Device. A helpful modern advancement tool that cautions individuals with or without hearing loss to make them aware of the existence of an environmental occurrence using auditory, visual, or tactile cues.

Amplitude. The maximum extent of a vibration or oscillation measured from the position of the equilibrium.

App/Application. An application, typically a small, specialized program downloaded onto computers and/or mobile devices.

Assistive. To give support or aid to; help; augment; enhance.

Assistive Listening Device (ALD). Any device that helps you overcome your hearing loss. Usually is applied to personal devices that transmit, process, or amplify sound, but usually not used to refer to hearing aids.

Assistive Technology (AT). A group of software or hardware devices by which people with disabilities can access computers. Can be specifically developed and marketed devices of off-the-shelf products that have been modified.

Audio. Sound that has been recorded that can be transmitted or reproduced; relating to hearing or sound.

Audiology. The branch of science and medicine concerned with the sense of hearing and balance.

Audio Shoe. An external frequency-modulated (FM) receiver device that attaches to a variety of hearing aids and implantable devices. These audio shoes require a compatible microphone/transmitter. Also sometimes called an FM boot.

Auditory Brainstem Implant (ABI). An implantable device like a cochlear implant except that it bypasses the cochlea altogether and with electrode contacts that are implanted directly to the base of the brainstem.

Auditory Trainer. Obsolete term used previously to describe a frequency-modulated (FM) hearing assistive technology (HAT) with microphone/transmitter and receiver, which also served as a hearing aid.

Augmentative and Alternative Communication (AAC). All nonoral forms of communication that are used to express thoughts, needs, wants, and ideas.

Auscultation. The method of listening to the sounds of the body.

Automatic Speech Recognition (ASR) Technology. Computer translation of spoken words into text.

Autophone. Automatic telephone detection feature of a hearing aid.

Autotelecoil. A feature of hearing aids that picks up a signal from a compatible telephone so that the hearing aid wearer can listen to the telephone without feedback.

Background Noise. See *Noise.*

Behind-the-Ear (BTE) Hearing Aids. A hearing aid that sits behind the ear with a tube connecting to an earpiece (earmold) that transmits amplified sound waves into the ear canal.

Biopsychosocial Model of Disability. A model of disability integrating the biological, psychological, and social aspects of a disability.

Bluetooth. A secure, short-range, wireless communication over the ISM band for devices such as smart devices, televisions, mobile phones, and so forth.

Bluetooth Low Energy (LE). Version of Bluetooth technology which allows for less energy consumption, compared to standard Bluetooth-enabled devices.

Bluetooth Streamer. See *Streamer.*

Bone-Anchored Hearing Aid. See *Bone-Anchored Implant.*

Bone-Anchored Implant (BAI). Surgically implanted hearing aid device that is based on bone conduction transmission.

Bone Conduction. Transmission of sound to the inner ear through the bones in the skull.

Brownian Motion. Random movement of particles in a medium.

Captioning. See *Text Interpreting.*

Channel. In a band of frequencies, pertains to using a limited portion of the frequency band to transmit information.

Closed Captions (CC). Process of displaying speech as text on a television or comparable display screen. See also *Text Interpreting.*

Cochlear Implant. A device that is surgically implanted into a person's cochlea to stimulate the auditory nerve to allow hearing to take place.

Communication Access Realtime Translation (CART). Also called open captioning or real-time stenography, or simply real-time captioning, is the general name of the system that court reporters, closed captioners and voice writers, and others use to convert speech to text. A trained operator uses keyboard or stenography methods to transcribe spoken speech into written text.

Compensatory strategies. An approach that may be environmental or behavioral that is used by a person to bypass a deficit in a particular area.

Condensation. Areas in which molecules are densely packed.

Conductive Hearing Loss (CHL). Physical anomaly or damage to the outer or middle ear that obstructs and attenuates sound transmitted to an otherwise normal inner ear.

Datalogging. The use of a computer to collect and analyze data, and to save and output the results of the analysis.

Decibel (dB). A scale used to describe the intensity of sound; 1/10 of a bel; a logarithmic scale; used in many forms of sound measurement and hearing tests.

Designated Interpreter. A specialized interpreter who works for the same individual or group in a repetitive way or over a long period of time, often becoming part of a team in a symbiotic working relationship.

Digital Enhanced Cordless Telecommunications (DECT) Technology. Wireless technology using the 1.9 GHz band, typically used with cordless phones.

Digital Enhanced Cordless Telecommunications (DECT) Ultra Low Energy (ULE) Technology. Version of DECT technology which allows for less energy consumption, compared to standard DECT devices.

Direct Audio Input (DAI). A feature on some hearing aids and implantable devices, which allows an external source to bypass the microphone via a hardwired connection. Example: Direct audio input to a hearing aid or implantable device from a portable music player (MP3) with a special cable.

Elasticity. The ability of an object or material to resume its normal shape after being compressed; the measure of stiffness of an object or material.

Electromagnetic Interference (EMI). Disturbance that affects an electrical circuit due to either electromagnetic induction or electromagnetic radiation emitted from an external source.

Electromagnetic Radiation (EMR). A kind of radiation that includes visible light, radio waves, gamma rays, and x-rays, in which electric and magnetic fields vary simultaneously; wireless hearing assistive technologies use certain frequency bands on the EM radiation spectrum.

FlashVP6. A proprietary video codec (file) developed by On2 Technologies that is used in Adobe Flash Player 8 and newer versions.

FM Boot. See *Audio Shoe.*

Frequency. The rate at which a vibration occurs that constitutes a wave, either in a material (as in sound waves), or in an electromagnetic field (as in radio waves and light), usually measured per second.

Frequency Hopping Spread Spectrum (FHSS) Technology. Wireless technology in which the transmission frequencies are determined by a spreading, or hopping, code. The receiver must be set to the same hopping code and must listen to the incoming signal at the right time and correct frequency in order to properly receive the signal.

Frequency Lowering. A way of increasing the access to high-frequency sounds, by digital manipulation, to a lower-frequency range where sounds are more likely to be audible.

Frequency Modulation (FM). A way of encoding signals over an alternating current wave through forced change in frequency; the manner of transmission for some hearing assistive technologies (HATs).

Giant Magnetoresistor (GMR). An electronic component that produces a large change in resistance of a conducting layer. "Giant" refers to its very large electrical signal. GMR is used in hearing aids with autotelecoils.

Global System for Mobile (GSM) Communications Technology. An open, digital cellular technology that transmits voice and data services for mobile devices over the 900 MHz band.

H.264. See *MPEG-4.*

Head Shadow Effect. A region of reduced amplitude of a sound in one ear because it is obstructed by the head. The obstruction caused by the head can account for a significant attenuation of overall intensity as well as cause a filtering effect.

Hearing Aid. An electroacoustic device that is designed to amplify sound for the wearer. The aim of these medical, FDA-regulated devices is to make speech more intelligible, and to correct impaired hearing as measured by audiometry.

Hearing Aid Compatibility (HAC). Usually used in reference to telephones, HAC ensures that a device provides internal means for effective use with hearing aids.

Hearing Assistive Technology (HAT). Devices that can help individuals with hearing loss function better in day-to-day situations, especially for communication and environmental awareness. HATs can be used with or without hearing aids or cochlear implants to make hearing easier.

Hearing Level (HL). The intensity of a sound measured in decibels with reference to audiometric zero and used to describe hearing sensitivity at specific test frequencies.

Hearing Loop. See *Induction Loop.*

High Frequency Average (HFA). An American National Standards Institute (ANSI) standard measurement regarding an average output (in dB SPL) for the amplitude-frequency response of a hearing aid at 1000, 1600, and 2500 Hz.

Implantable Device. Implantable hearing device examples include cochlear implants (CIs), auditory brainstem implants (ABIs), bone-anchored implant/bone-anchored hearing aids (BAIs/BAHAs), and middle ear implants (MEIs).

Individualized Education Program (IEP). Mandated by the Individuals with Disabilities Education Act (IDEA), an IEP defines a plan of individual objectives for a child with special needs and is designed to help children reach educational goals more easily than they otherwise would.

Induction. As in electromagnetic induction, it is the production of an electromotive force across a conductor when it is exposed to a varying magnetic field; the manner of transmission for some hearing assistive technologies (HATs).

Induction Loop. A method of wireless transmission of a signal to a hearing aid or other assistive device via a loop of wire around a room, building, vehicle, or other selected area. This can also be incorporated into neckloops, behind-the-ear silhouettes, kiosks, and countertop units.

Induction Neckloop. See *Induction Loop.*

Induction Silhouette. See *Induction Loop.*

Inductive Coupling. Describes the use of a telecoil to pick up the transmission of speech and other desirable sounds via electromagnetic induction. See also *Induction,* *Induction Loop,* and *Telecoil.*

Industrial, Scientific, and Medical (ISM) Frequency Band. Typically thought of as the 2.4 GHz range of radio frequencies designated for the transmission of devices used in industry, science, and medicine.

Information Technology (IT). The application of computers and telecommunications equipment to store, retrieve, transmit, and manipulate data, often in the context of a business or other enterprise. Typically refers to computers and computer networks.

Infrared (IR). Invisible radiant energy, electromagnetic radiation with longer wavelengths than those of visible light, extending from the nominal red edge of the visible spectrum; the manner of transmission for some hearing assistive technologies (HATs).

Instant Messaging (IM). A type of online chat that offers real-time text transmission over the Internet.

Intensity. Sound power per unit area. Sound intensity is not the same physical quantity as sound pressure. Hearing is directly sensitive to sound pressure which is related to sound intensity.

Internet. A global system of interconnected computer networks that uses the standard Internet protocol suite (TCP/IP) to link several billion devices worldwide.

Internet of Things (IoT). The connection between multiple wireless devices, such as a piconet, in which at least one device has the capacity to connect to the Internet.

In-the-Ear (ITE) Hearing Aids. A hearing aid that sits within the ear canal and transmits amplified sound waves into the ear canal.

Inverse Square Law. States that the intensity of a sound is inversely proportional to the square of the distance that the sound has traveled.

Lipreading. Technique of understanding speech by visually interpreting the movement of the lips, face, and tongue when normal sound is not available, relying also on information provided by the context, knowledge of the language, and any residual hearing.

Local Area Network (LAN). Computer network that interconnects computers within a limited area such as a home, school, computer lab, or office building using network media.

Locus of Control. Refers to the extent to which individuals believe they can control events affecting them.

Long-Term Evolution (LTE). A wireless broadband technology designed to support roaming Internet access via mobile phones and handheld devices.

Loudspeaker. An electroacoustic transducer; a device that converts an electrical audio signal into a corresponding sound.

Mapping/MAP. Term used to describe programming of an implantable device such as a cochlear implant and auditory brainstem implant using electrical stimulation of neural tissue.

Masking. Occurs when the perception of one sound is affected by the presence of another sound.

Medical Model of Disability. A sociopolitical model by which illness or disability, being the result of a physical condition intrinsic to the individual, may reduce the individual's quality of life and cause clear disadvantages to the individual.

Microphone. An acoustic-to-electric transducer or sensor that converts soundwaves in the air to an electrical signal.

Middle Ear Implant (MEI). Surgically implanted hearing aid connected to or partially located in the middle ear to amplify vibrations into the inner ear.

Mixed Hearing Loss (MHL). Hearing loss that is the combination of both conductive hearing loss and sensorineural hearing loss.

MP3. Also known as "MPEG" or the Motion Picture Experts group; is an audio coding format for digital audio which uses a form of data compression.

MPEG-4. A digital multimedia format most commonly used to store video and audio, but can also be used to store other data such as subtitles and still images.

M-Ratings. A hearing aid compatibility rating between a hearing aid microphone and a mobile phone.

Near Field Communication (NFC) Technology. A form of short-range wireless communication where the antenna used is much smaller than the wavelength of the carrier signal.

Needs Assessment. A systematic process for determining and addressing needs, or "gaps" between current conditions and desired conditions or "wants." The discrepancy between the current condition and wanted condition must be measured to appropriately identify the need.

Noise. An aperiodic complex signal. May be used to describe any undesirable signal, whether acoustic, electric, magnetic, or biologic; in the case of hearing, background noise obscures or masks speech sounds making it more difficult to perceive.

Open Captions (OC). A text display of all of the words and sounds heard during a production presented on a screen for visual media; a nonbroadcasted signal that is always present on the screen and cannot be turned off.

Outcome Measures. The assessment of the benefits of an intervention such as amplification or the goals and objectives that are established after the initial diagnostic workup of a client.

Participation Restriction. A problem experienced by an individual in involvement in life situations.

Personal Sound Amplification Product (PSAP). Wearable electronic products that are intended to amplify sounds for people who do not have hearing loss.

Piconet. Small network of wireless devices, which become an Internet of Things (IoT) if connected to the Internet.

Public Address System. An electronic sound amplification and distribution system with a microphone, amplifier, and loudspeakers, used to allow a person to address a large group.

Quality of Life (QoL). An indicator of the general well-being of a person.

Radio Frequency (RF) Interference. See *Electromagnetic Interference (EMI).*

Receiver. An electronic device that receives signals wirelessly from a microphone transmitter (e.g., FM receiver); in hearing aids it is an electronic component that refers to the miniature loudspeaker that delivers the previously amplified sound into the ear canal.

Receiver In-the-Canal/Receiver In-the-Ear (RITE) Hearing Aids. A hearing aid in which the receiver is inside the ear canal and connected to a behind-the-ear (BTE) hearing aid via thin tubing; the BTE unit is particularly small, lightweight, and inconspicuous.

Reference Test Gain (RTG). An American National Standards Institute (ANSI) standard measurement regarding the gain (output) of a hearing aid when the gain control is adjusted such that a 60 dB SPL input signal provides a high-frequency average (HFA) value that is 17 dB below the HFA at a 90 dB input SPL (OSPL90) value. In this book, RTG is used to help derive the RSETS and RTLS values for telecoil sensitivity.

Relative Stimulation Equivalent Telephone Sensitivity (RSETS). An American National Standards Institute (ANSI) standard measurement regarding telecoil performance in hearing aids with regard to telephones; specifically this is a difference measure comparing the high-frequency average (HFA) of the telecoil response to microphone response and ideally should yield an RSETS value of 0.

Relative Test Loop Sensitivity (RTLS). An American National Standards Institute (ANSI) standard measurement regarding telecoil performance in hearing aids receptive to electromagnetic energy sources, particularly an induction loop; specifically this is a difference measure comparing the high-frequency average (HFA) of the telecoil response to microphone response and ideally should yield an RTLS value of 0.

Reliability. Indicator of finding replicable results upon repeated operations.

Remote Microphone. A microphone without a physical cable connecting it directly to the amplifying equipment with which it is associated; typically associated with hearing aids and implantable devices.

Reverberation. The interpretation of the persistence of sound after a sound is produced.

RT60. The time required for reflections of a direct sound to decay 60 dB.

Self-Efficacy. One's belief in one's own ability to complete task or goal.

Sensorineural Hearing Loss (SNHL). Damage to the inner ear and/or auditory nerve that results in hearing loss.

Service Animal. Animal, usually a dog, that has been specially trained to perform tasks to assist people with disabilities.

Service Dog. A type of service dog specifically selected and trained to assist individuals with hearing loss by alerting them to important sounds, such as doorbells, smoke alarms, ringing telephones, or alarm clocks. They may also work outside the home, alerting to such sounds such as sirens, forklifts, and a person calling the handler's name.

Short Message Service (SMS). Text messaging service component of phone, Web, or mobile communication system.

Signaling Device. See *Alerting Device*.

Signal-to-Noise Ratio (SNR). Measure that compares the level of desired signal to the level of background noise. A positive decibel (dB) value indicates that the speech is louder than the noise, whereas a negative dB value indicates that the noise is louder than speech.

Social Model of Disability. States that disability is caused by the way society is organized, rather than by a person's impairment or difference.

Soundfield. Refers to the use of loudspeakers as opposed to headphones to transmit sound.

Sound Level Meter. Instrument that measures sound pressure level (SPL).

Sound Pressure Level (SPL). Measure of the sound pressure of a specific sound relative to a reference value; measured in dB.

Sound Pressure Level Inductive Telephone Simulation (SPLITS). An American National Standards Institute (ANSI) standard measurement regarding telecoil performance in hearing aids with regard to telephones; specifically this is an output measure comparing the high-frequency average (HFA) of the telecoil response to microphone response and used to determine RSETS.

Sound Pressure Level Inductive Vertical Field (SPLIV). An American National Standards Institute (ANSI) standard measurement regarding telecoil performance in hearing aids receptive to electromagnetic energy sources, particularly an induction loop; specifically this is an output measure comparing the high-frequency average (HFA) of the telecoil response to microphone response and used to determine RTLS.

Speechreading. Lipreading in order to determine the intended meaning of a speaker.

Speech Therapy. Training to help people with speech, language, or articulation deficits.

Stenograph. Keyboard instrument used to record phonetic or arbitrary symbols.

Stenotype. Instrument that is used to record speech in syllables or phonemes.

Stethoscope. Acoustic or electroacoustic instrument for listening to someone's heart or breathing.

Streamer. A device that provides one-way communication, or a stream of data, to a wireless device.

Subtitles. Nonbroadcasted captions displayed that translate or transcribe the dialogue or narrative.

Telecoil. Supplemental input device for a hearing aid; small coil of wire around a core that will induce an electric current in the coil when it is in the presence of a changing magnetic field; for use with telephones and other audio devices.

Telecommunication Device for the Deaf (TDD). See *Teletypewriter*.

Telecommunications. Communication at a distance by technical means, particularly through electromagnetic transmission.

Telecommunications Relay Service (TRS). Operating system that allows those who are hard of hearing or deaf to call a standard telephone via an assistive telecommunication device, such as TTY, VCO, captioned phone, or videophone.

Teletypewriter (TTY). An electromechanical typewriter that can receive and send typed messages from point to point over various types of communication channels.

Texting/Text Messages. See *Short Message Service (SMS)*.

Text Interpreting. An electronic note-taking system designed to provide meaning-for-meaning, or verbatim, transcription of spoken English into text; service is provided by a trained provider using specialized hardware and software, and the output is displayed on a projection screen, laptop computer, or smart device.

Timbre. The quality of a sound or tone that distinguishes different types of sound production, such as voices or instruments.

Tinnitus. Disorder characterized by ringing or buzzing in the ears.

Transducer. Device that converts energy from one form to another; refers to a variety of microphones, headphones, loudspeakers, and so forth.

Transduction. Process of converting energy from one form of energy to another.

Transmitter. Electronic device that generates and amplifies a carrier wave for the purpose of transmitting to a receiver.

T-Ratings. A hearing aid compatibility rating for hearing aid telecoil and for mobile phones.

Turnkey System. An electronic device, such as a computer system, that has been customized for a particular application.

Ultraviolet (UV) Light. Electromagnetic radiation with a wavelength shorter than visible light but longer than X-rays.

Validity. The quality of being factually sound or logic; findings that truly represent the phenomenon you are claiming to measure.

Videophone. Telephone device transmitting and receiving a visual image as well as sound; a device for individuals who are deaf and hard of hearing to communicate with other videophone users, or to place a call to a relay operator via sign language.

Videotelephony. Telephone with a video display, capable of simultaneous video and auditory for communication between people in real time.

Voice Carry Over (VCO). Allows individuals with hearing loss who are able to speak to use their voice while receiving text-based responses from a person who is a hearing caller; a relay operator facilitates this type of telecommunication.

Voice over Internet Protocol (VoIP). A method of delivering audio and video over the Internet.

Wavelength. Distance from one point on a wave to another point of a periodic wave as it is traveling in a direction.

Wi-Fi. Local area wireless technology that allows an electronic device to exchange data, or connect to the Internet.

Index

Note: Page numbers in **bold** reference non-text material.